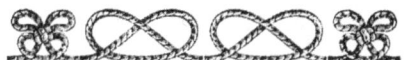

This book is dedicated to
Albertha Griffin Hull, my grandmother
Estelle Braithwaite McKorkle, my mother
and to
all of those strivers whose dreams were deferred.

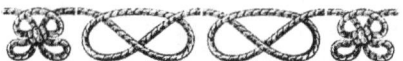

BRAID SCULPTURE
THE ART OF COMBLESS HAIRSTYLING
By Richelle Braithwaite

Published in 2009 by
The Riqui Lox System
www.riquilox.com
e-mail:riqui@riquilox.com

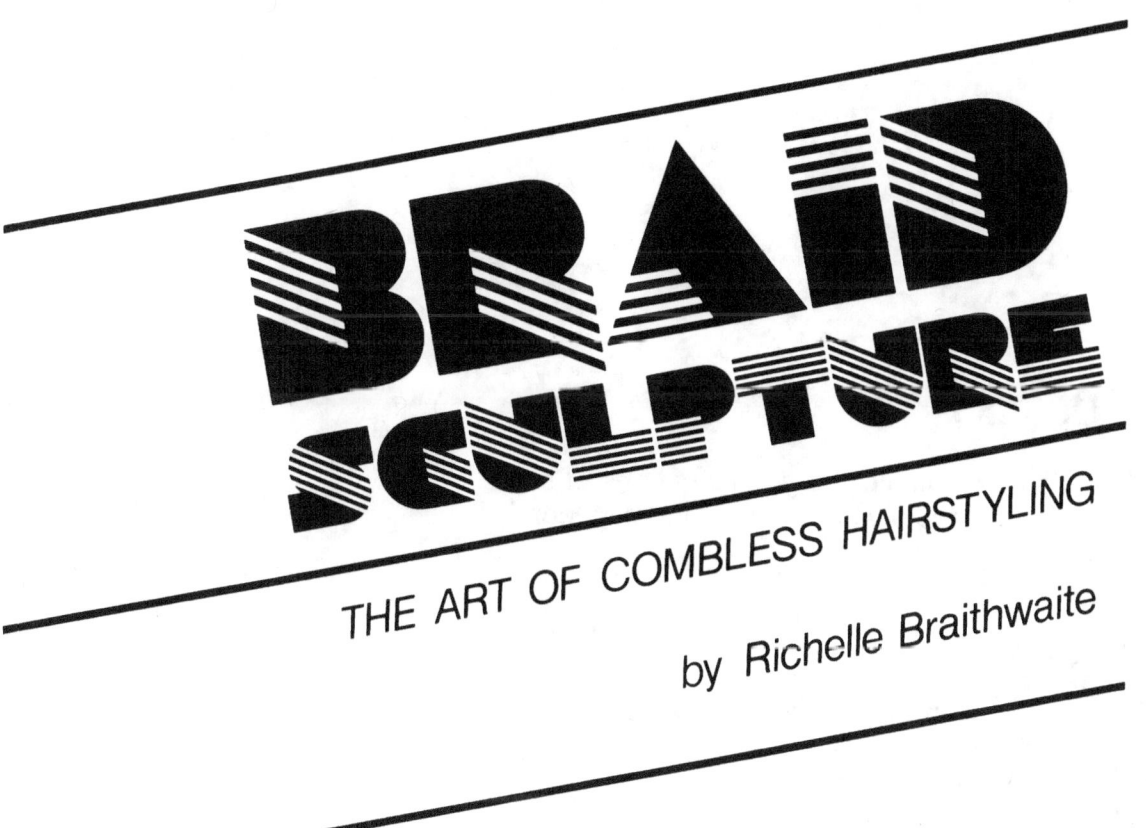

BRAID SCULPTURE

THE ART OF COMBLESS HAIRSTYLING

by Richelle Braithwaite

A MESSAGE FROM THE AUTHOR

"Every time I comb my hair it comes out by the handful!" This is the complaint of far too many Black women. Long, short, or medium lengths can all be nicely styled. But what of the woman whose hair is broken off at the back, the top, or the sides? What about chemically damaged hair, or the woman who wants her hair to return to its natural texture? Certain hair textures, in spite of being conditioned, suffer abuse from constant pressing, perming, curling, and combing. This book is a partial solution to these problems.

Why a book on braid hairstyling? One reason is for posterity, and another reason is to help fill the gap that exists in the methods of hairstyling. The models and I hope you enjoy the hair styles you find in this book and that you find some that suit your fancy.

—Richelle Braithwaite

GLOSSARY

The following definitions are explanations of some terms in the book with which you may not be familiar:

PLAITS
Also known as individual or single braids.

CORNROWS
When the hair is braided along the scalp in a continuous line, as in rows of corn.

TWISTS
An interlocking of the hair, using two strands.

EXTENSIONS
The adding of natural or synthetic materials to the hair in order to lengthen, thicken, or embellish it.

HUMAN HAIR
Used when curling is desired. Best results are obtained if the person's hair is permed, waved, or done in very small braids.

SYNTHETIC HAIR
Works well with natural, unpermed hair. Contrary to rumor, it does not cut the hair. It allows braids to be worn for a longer time.

ROLLS
Turning braids in on themselves to give height and width to a style.

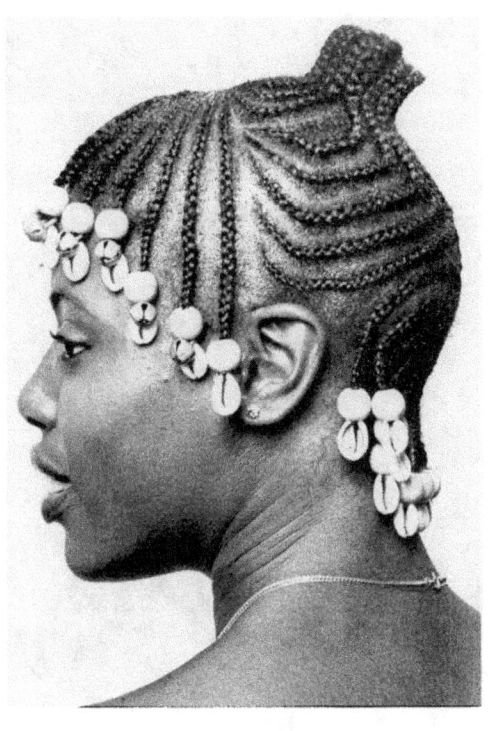

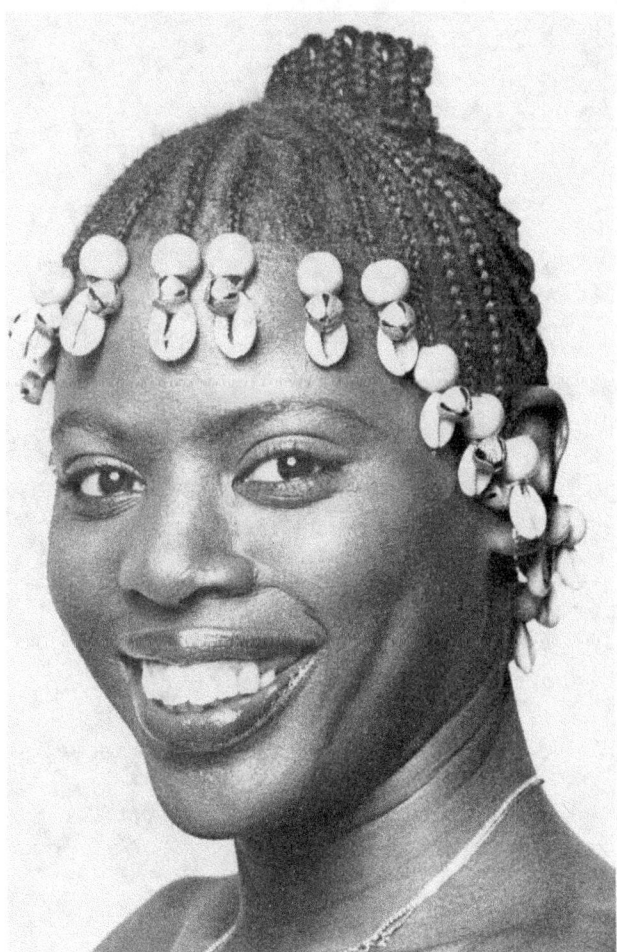

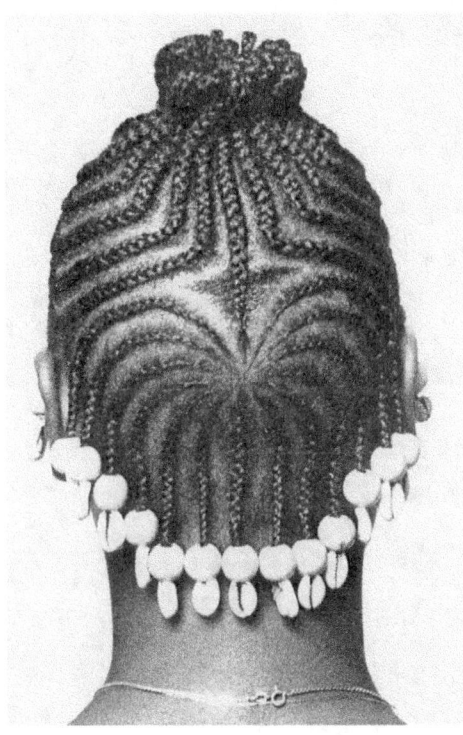

Beads, bells, and shells. Drucilla sports a cornrowed braid style, and its ornamentation accentuates the beauty of her face. The back view grabs the eye and makes its "point".

3

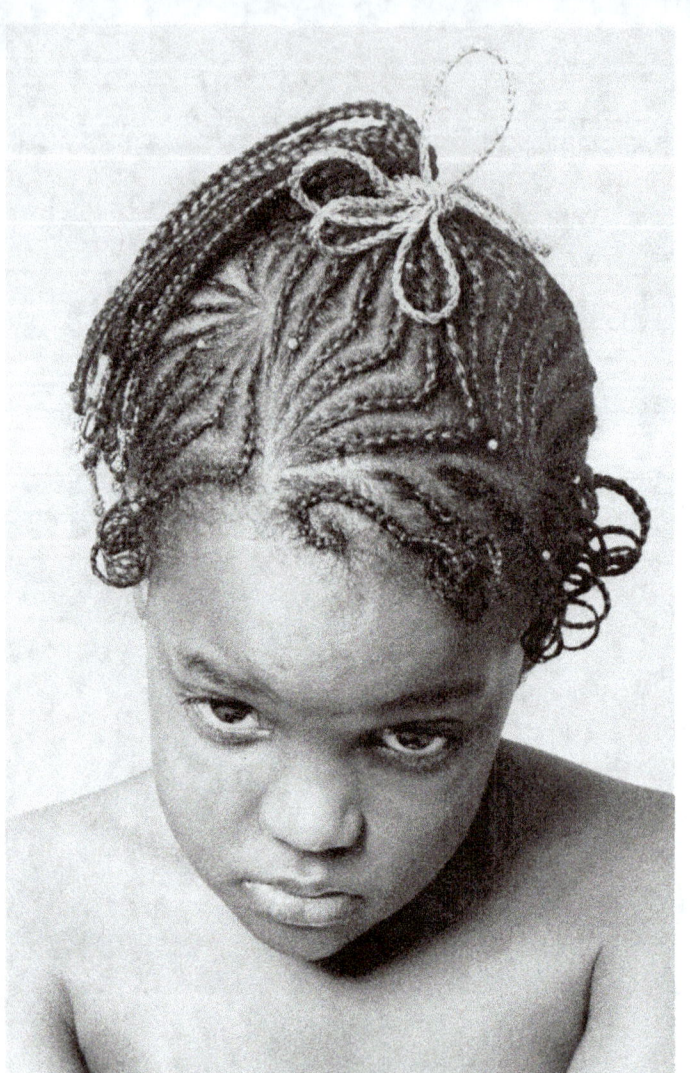

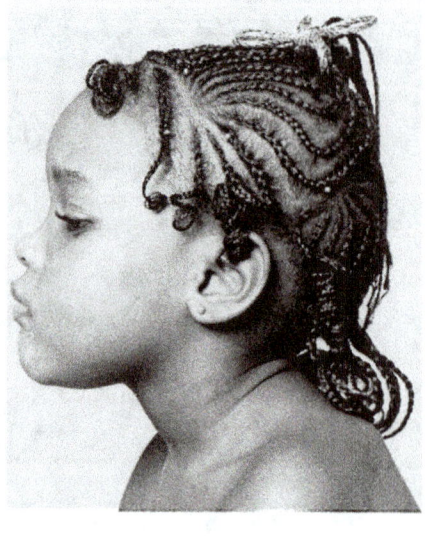

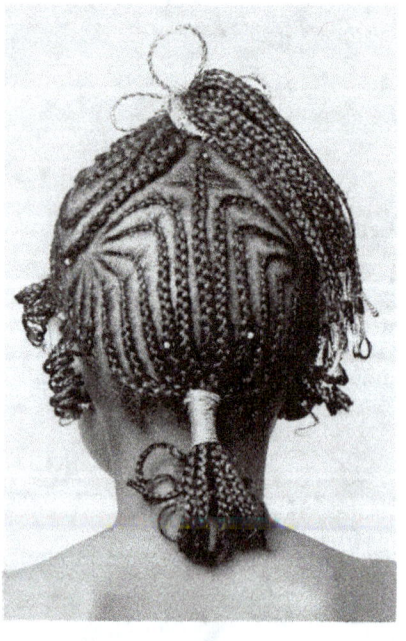

Little girl curls. Dakisha can charm any heart with her elfish sweetness. Here she wears a double-layered cornrowed style. The creative parting draws the eye to the decorative patterns and assures Dakisha of her share of compliments.

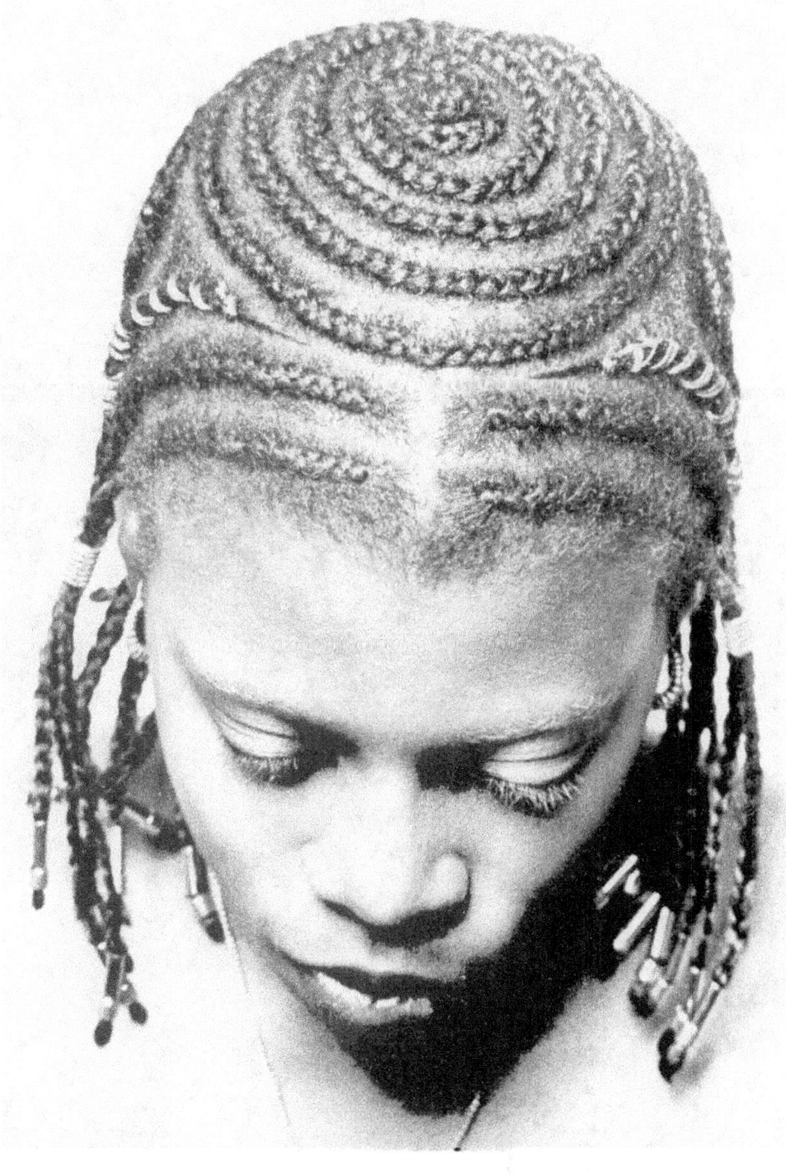

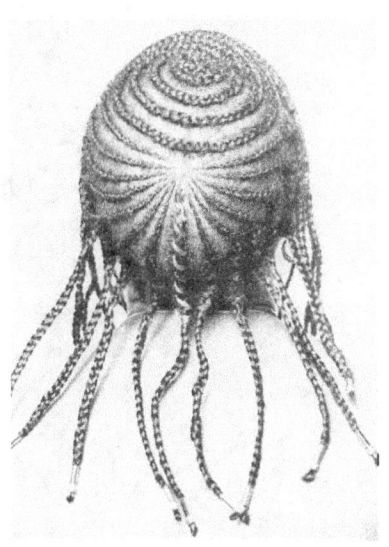

Diane's style incorporates both circular and angular motifs. The sunburst design topped by a spiral is of ancient origin and can be found in many different cultures.

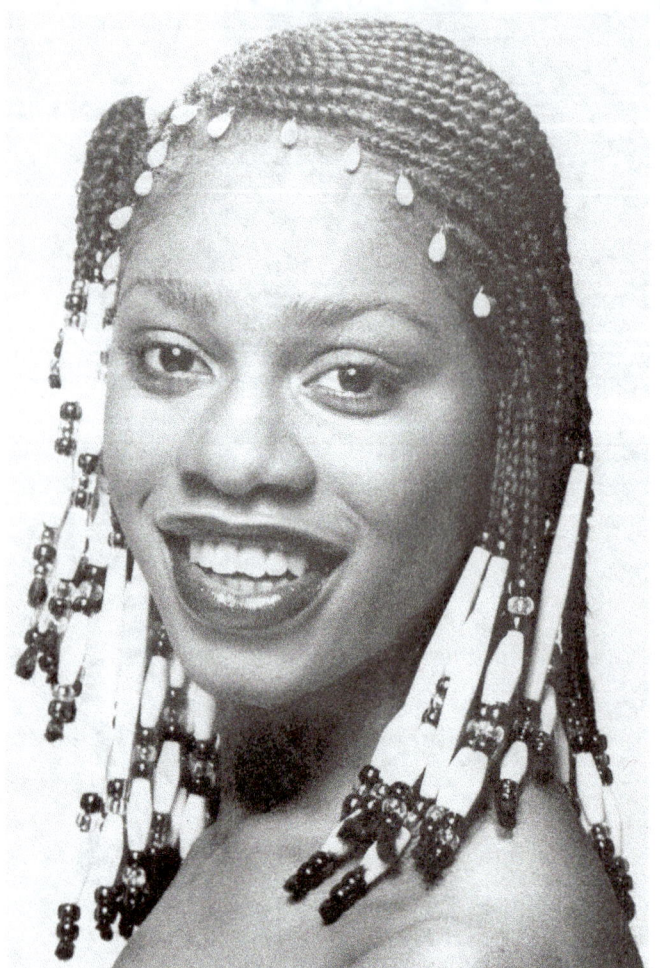

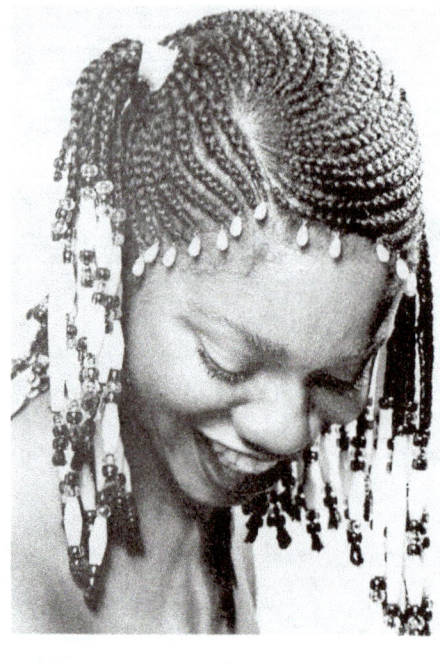

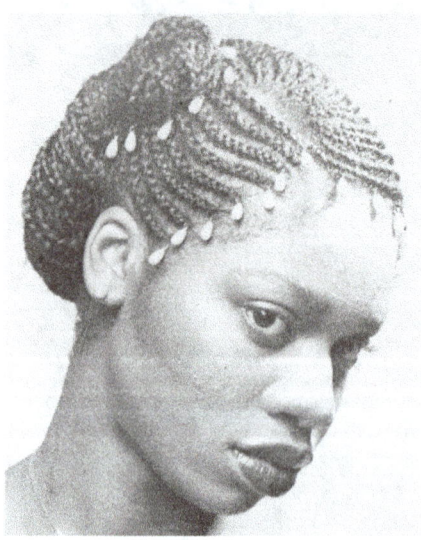

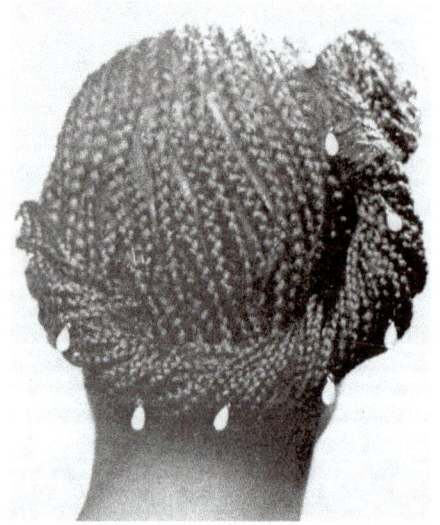

Casual and elegant. This beaded beauty
says it all. Marcia's multi-layered extension style lends itself to soft shapings.
The elegant alternate is a head-hugging
roll studded with pearls.

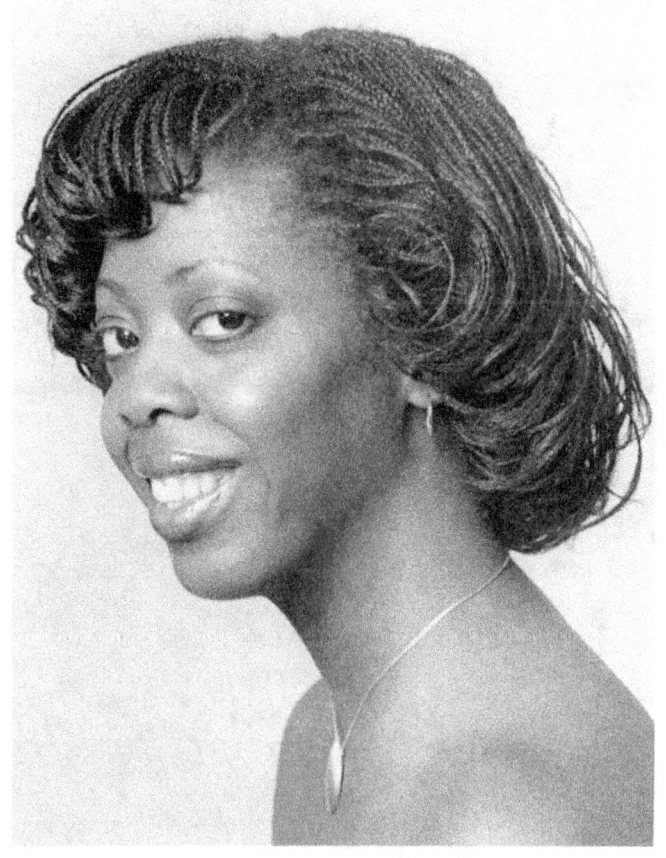

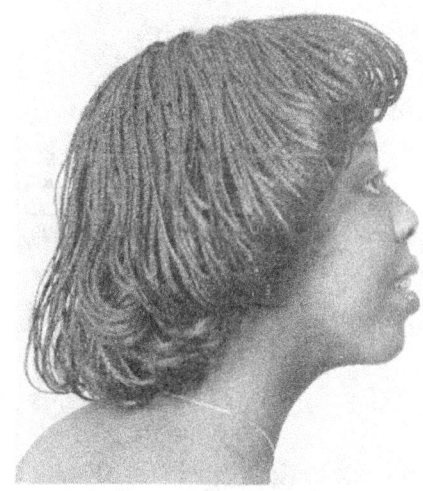

Richelle's own thick medium length hair is done up in hundreds of tiny single braids. This allows for a wide variety of styling, such as the "Jerri" curl when set on perm rods, or the crimped look when the style is wet, braided into six or seven large sections, dried and let loose.

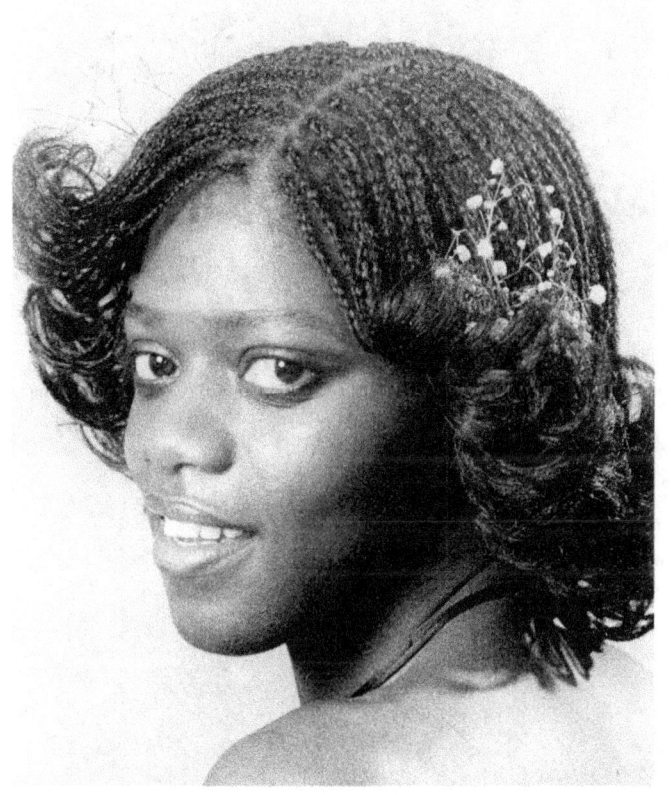

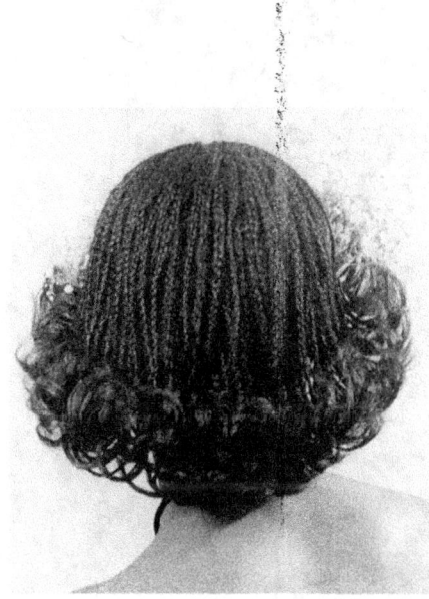

Moirelle's perky upturned 'do is made up of individual human hair extensions. The ends are left undone to create a fluffy effect when curled with thermal irons. An alternate style can be created by pulling the hair back from the face and securing it with a headband.

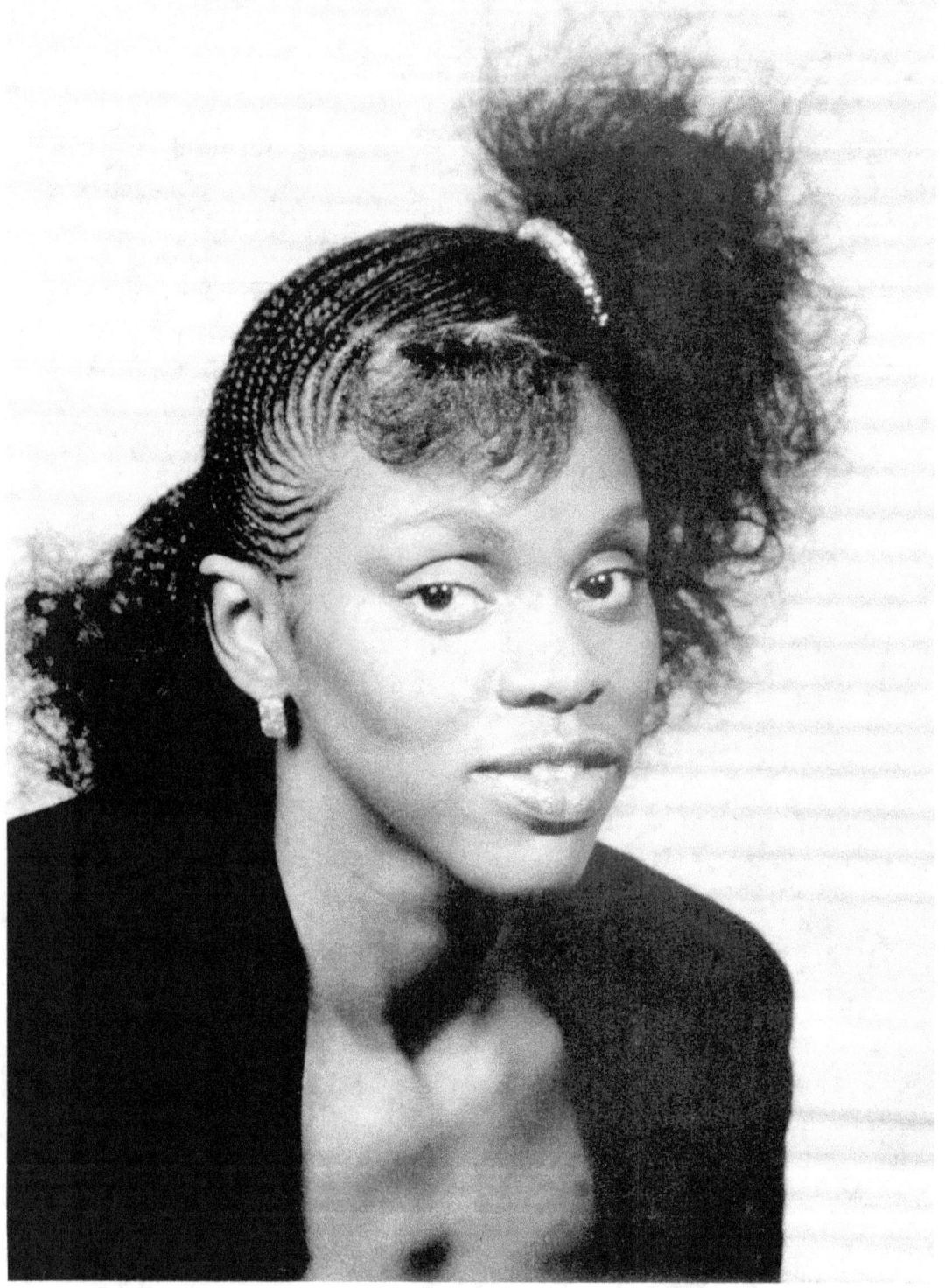

Once again shoulder length hair is styled to enhance the wearer's features. Leza's hair is multi-layered into a ponytail, with single braids in the back topped by another layer of cornrows. All of the ends are left undone so that curling will produce volume.

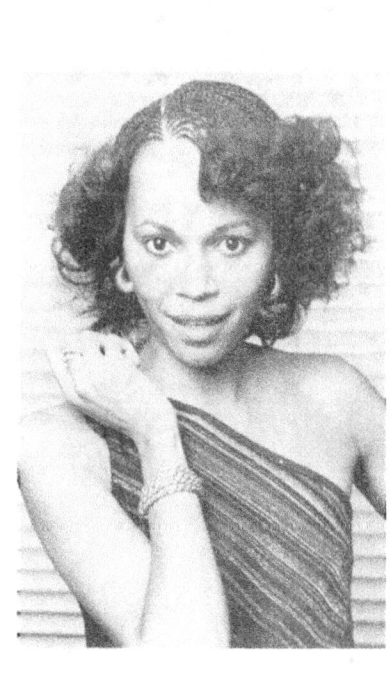

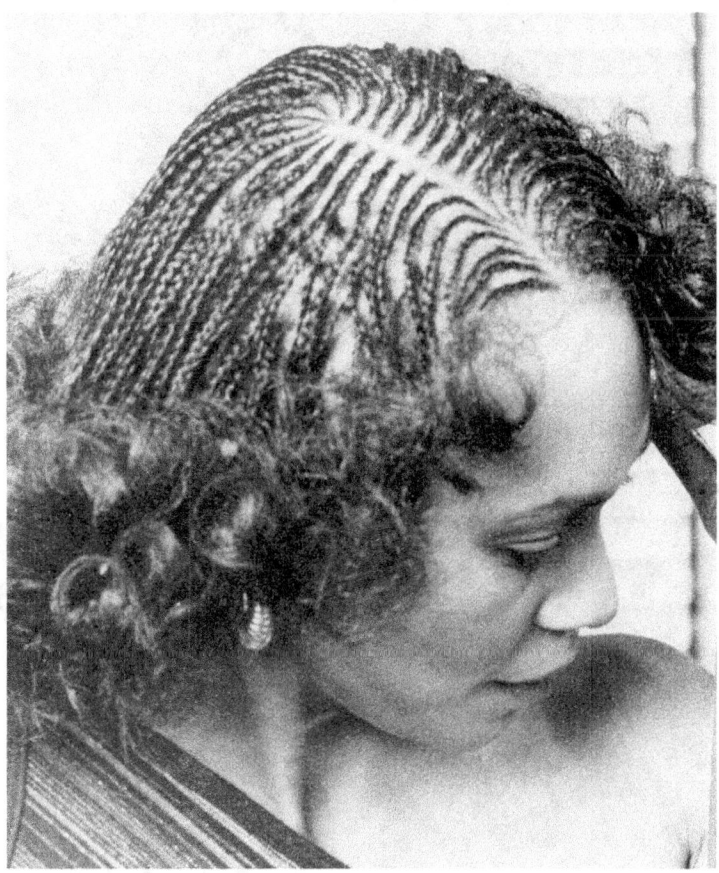

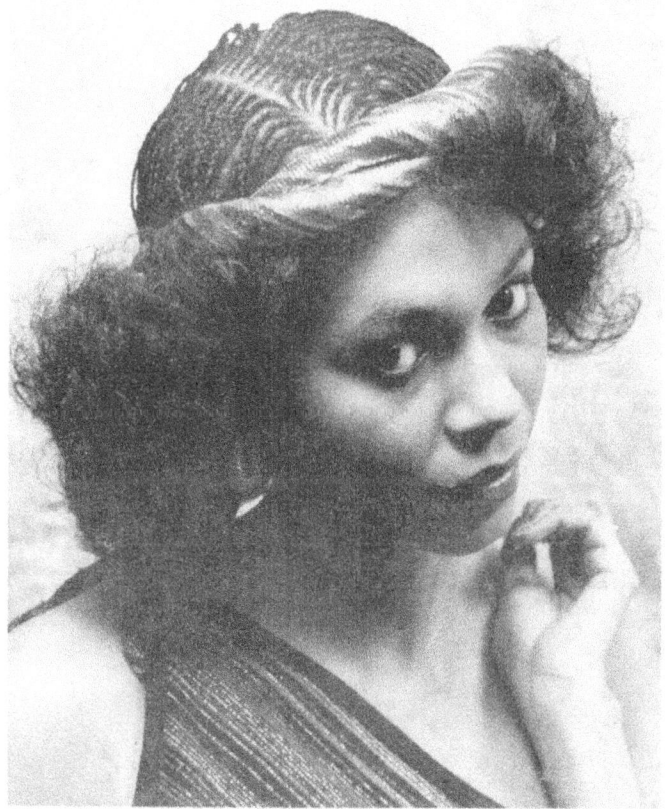

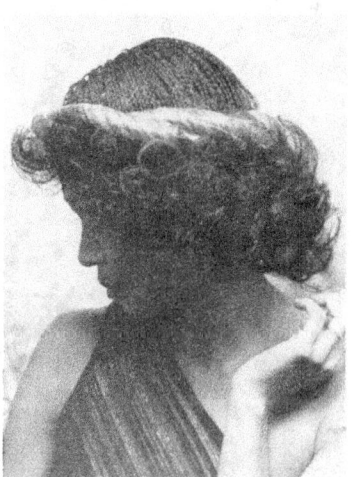

Alternate for a perm. Terri's permed hair is braided in individual plaits and is topped by a layer of tiny cornrows. The ends are left loose and then curled. For a more compact look, the hair is rolled around the head and ends in a curly bang.

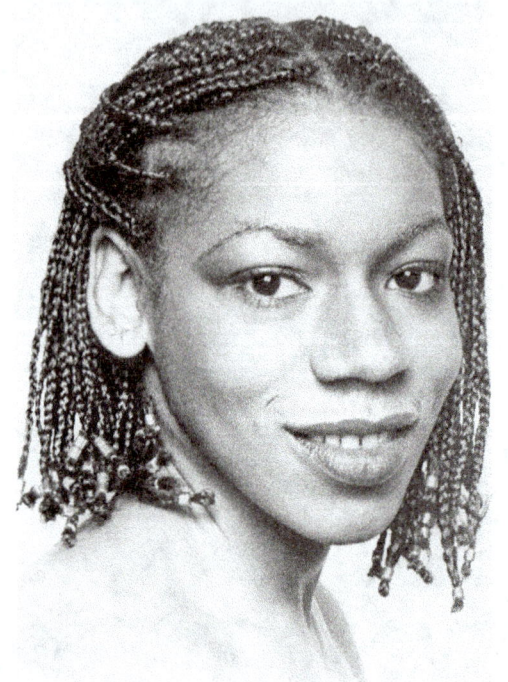
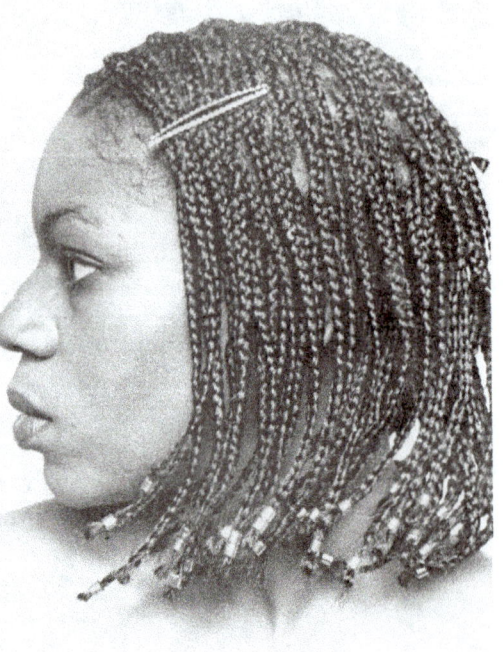

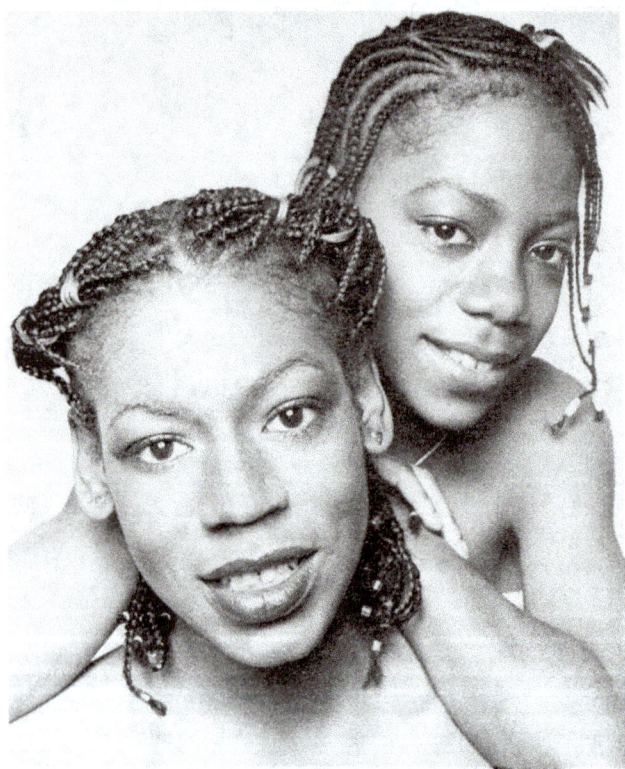

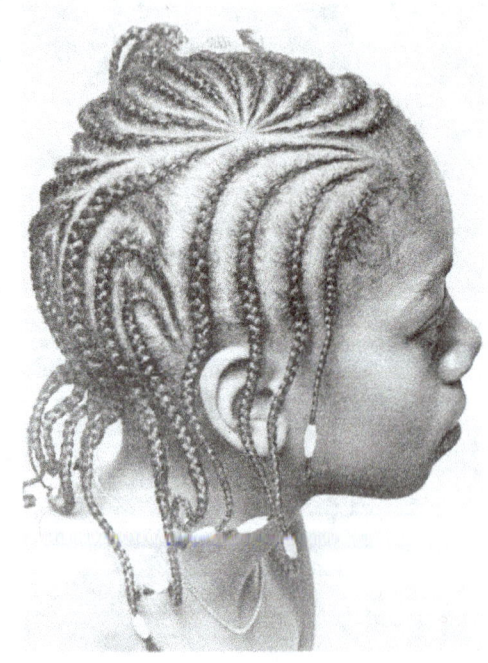

Mother and daughter. This individual plait style, done with synthetic hair, is very versatile, it can be worn hanging, rolled, or braided into two large cornrows. Jackie's daughter has her hair cornrowed in a style that has many "points" of interest.

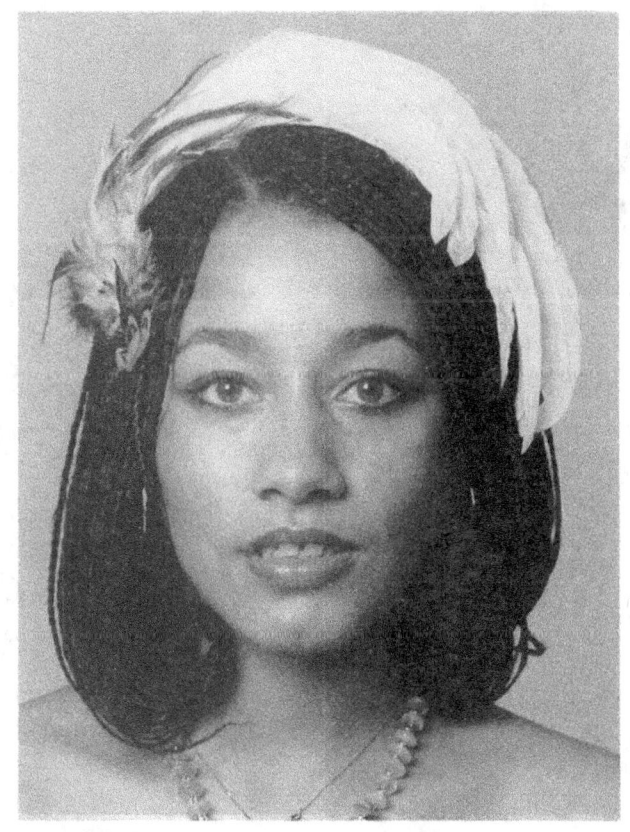

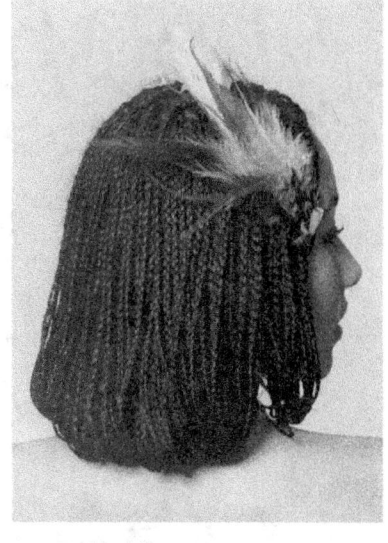

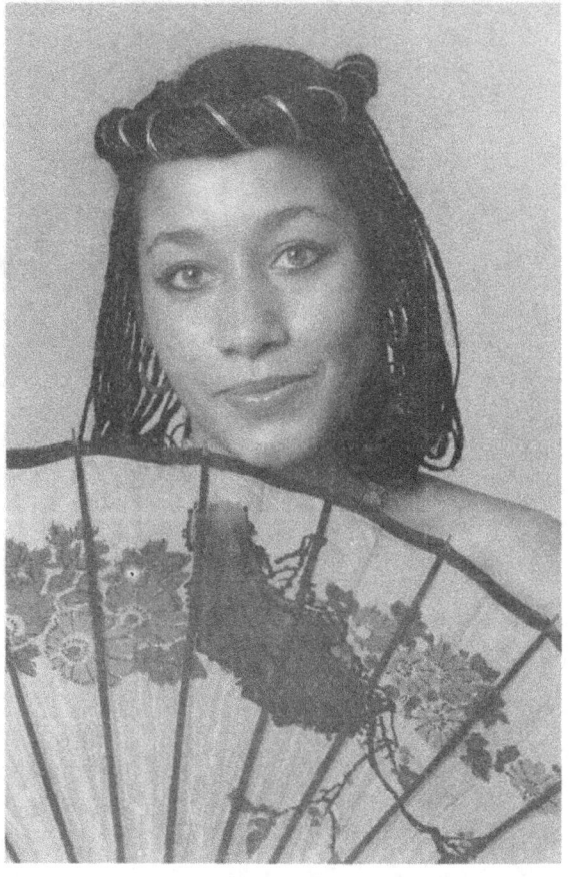

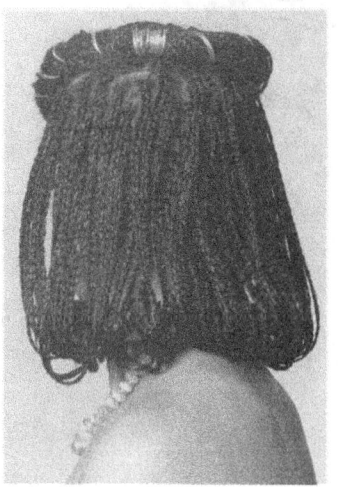

Bernadette's pageboy is of individual plaits done with human hair extensions. For an exotic effect, the braids are rolled around the top of the head in a crown and banded with gold thread. By sweeping all of the braids over to one side and curling them softly, an elegant alternate style can be created.

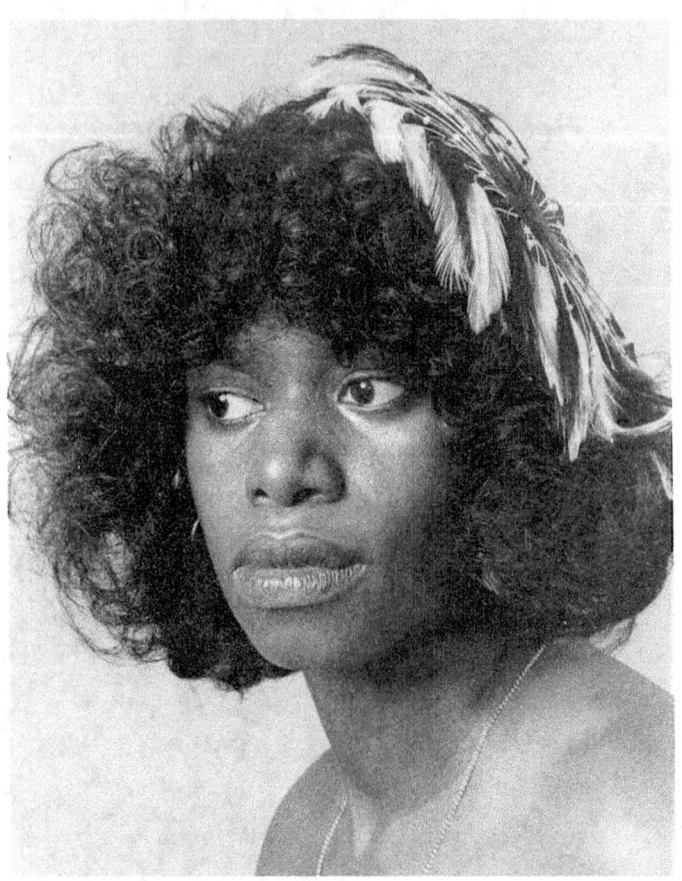

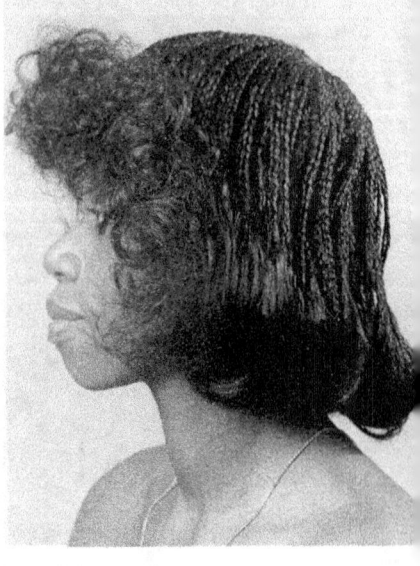

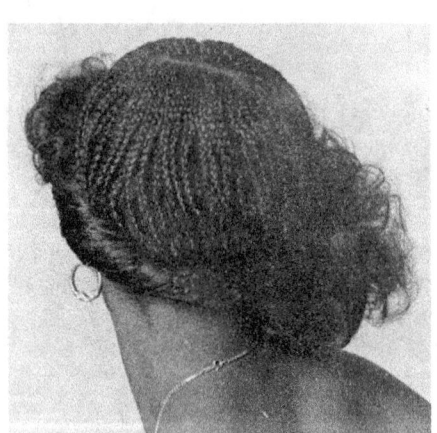

Is it or isn't it? Here is a style that requires a second look. Using human hair extensions, Denise's three layers of tiny cornrows are left open at the ends and curled to create their face framing design. A feathered swirl accents it. The alternate style is swept up off the neck. A third style can be created by ending the roll at the right eye.

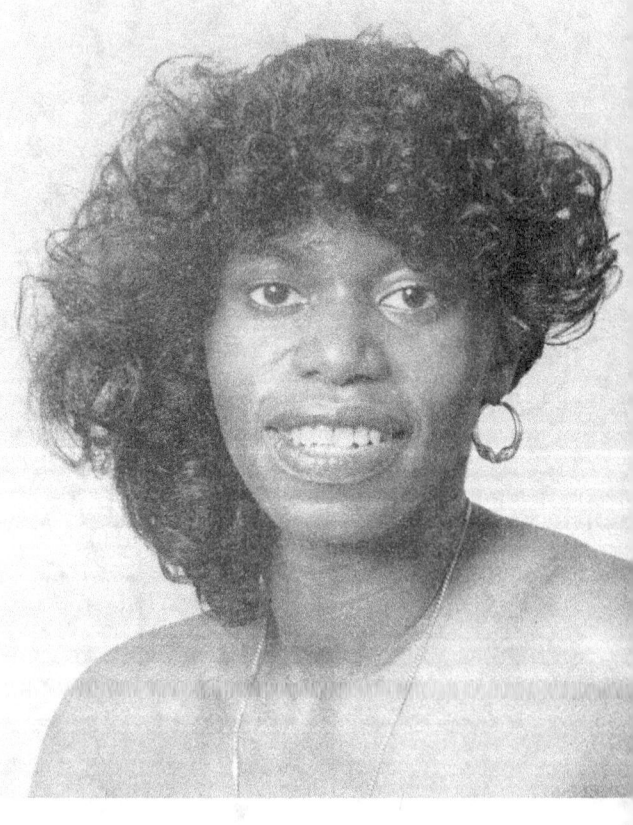

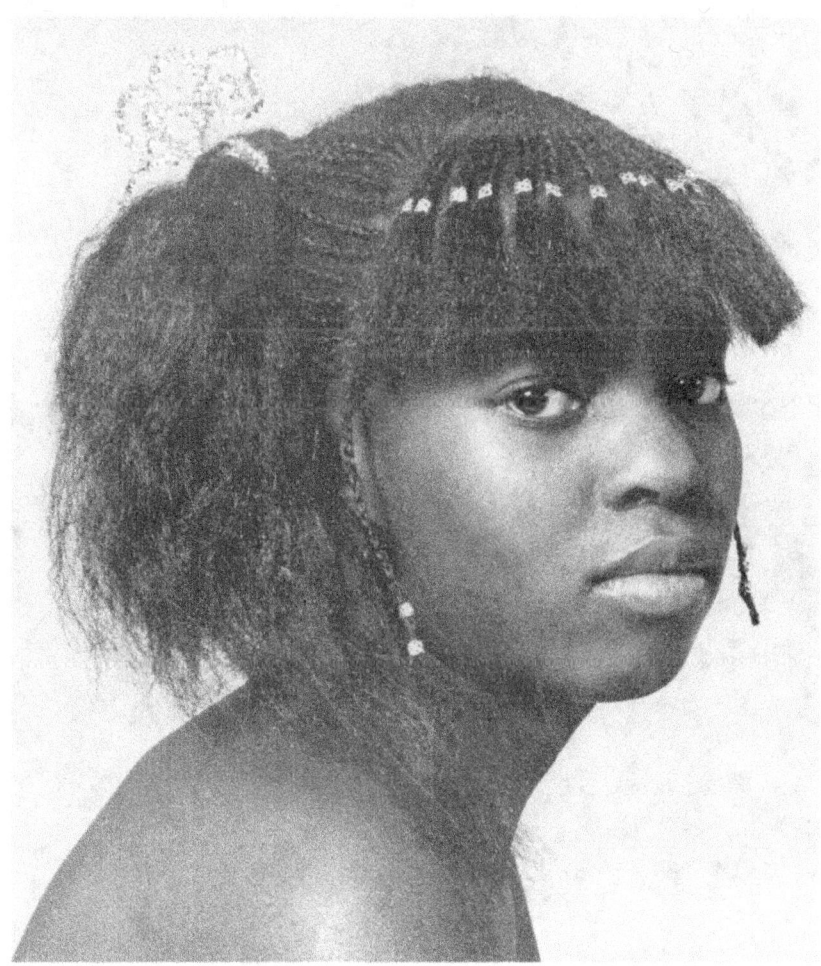

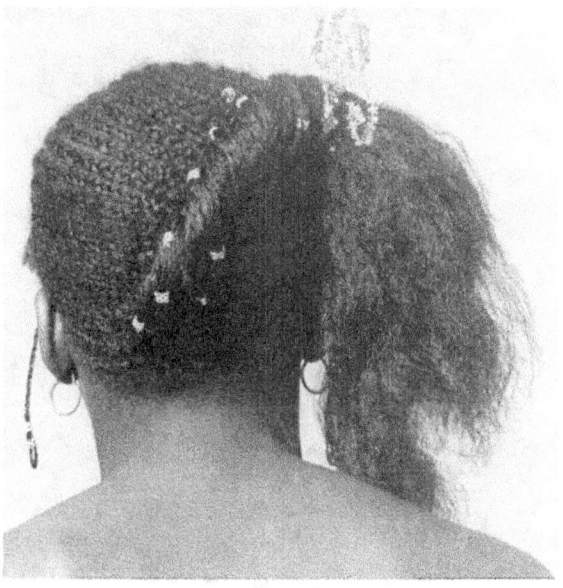

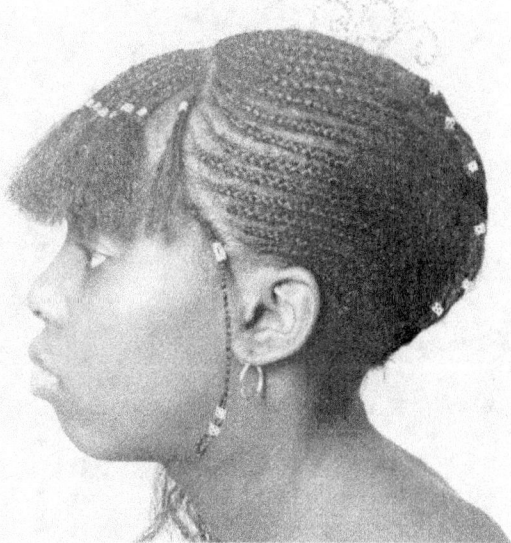

This young lady wears a side-directed ponytail wrapped in silver. This style works well with either type of extenions. For versatility, braid the hair down from the crown to the nape of the neck.

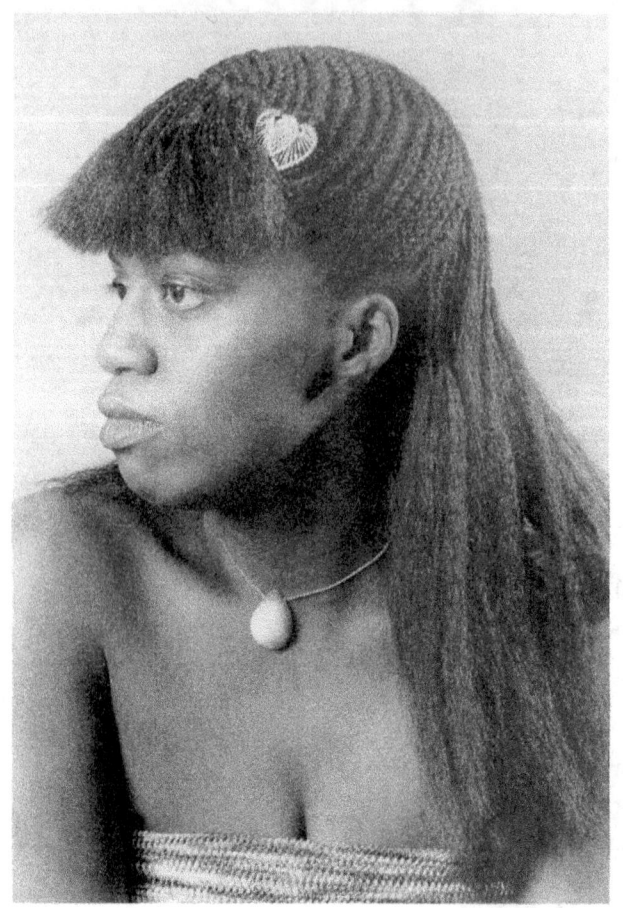

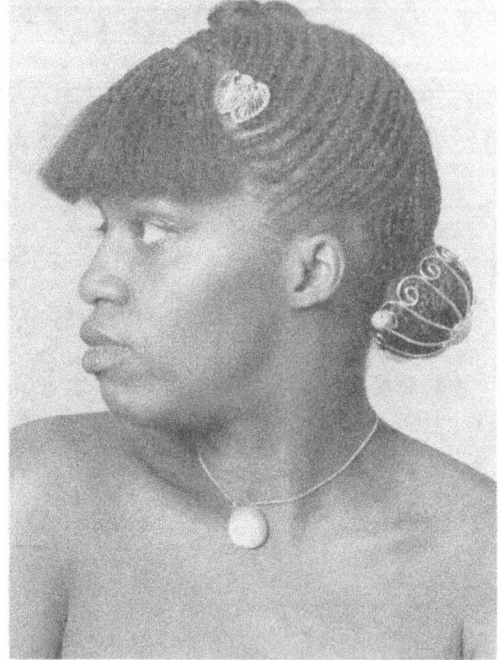

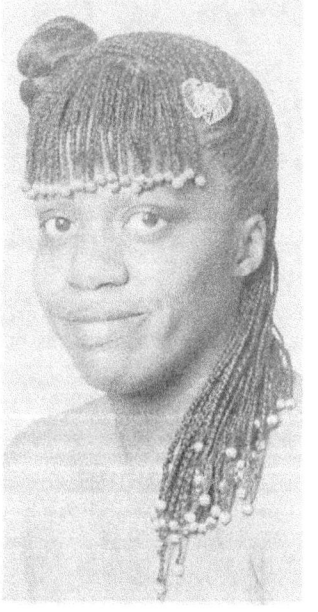

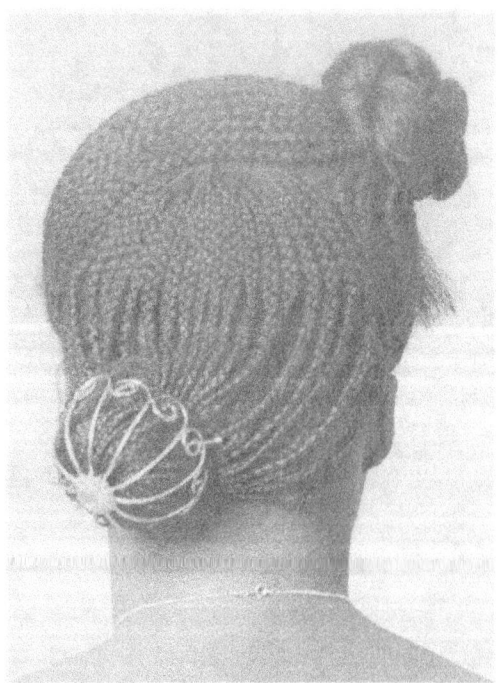

Lillian lets it all hang loose and fluffy. If
wild and free isn't your style, try these
two loveknots. If beads are more to
your liking, you can see how easily this
style accommodates you. Enjoy!

14

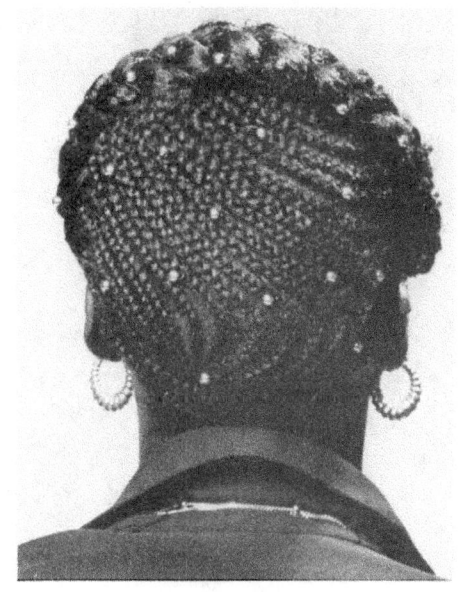

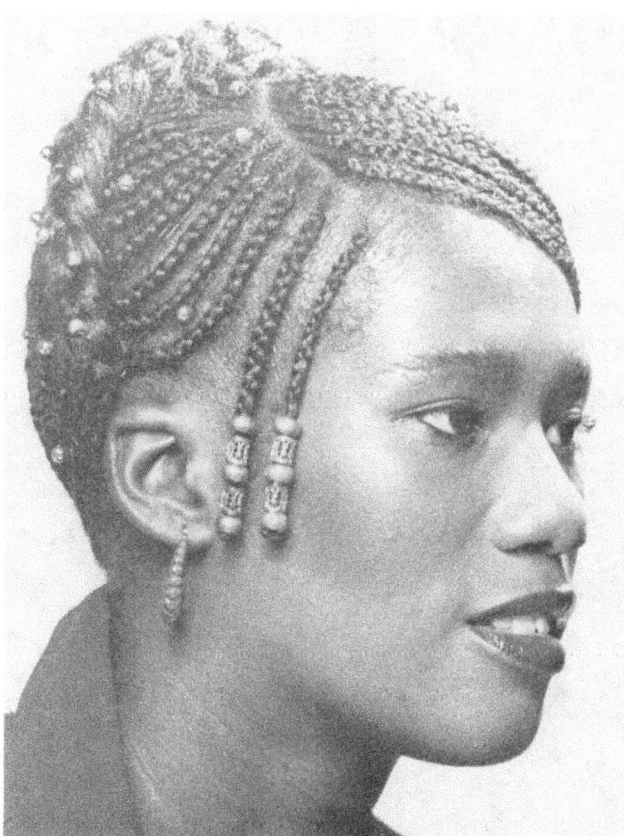

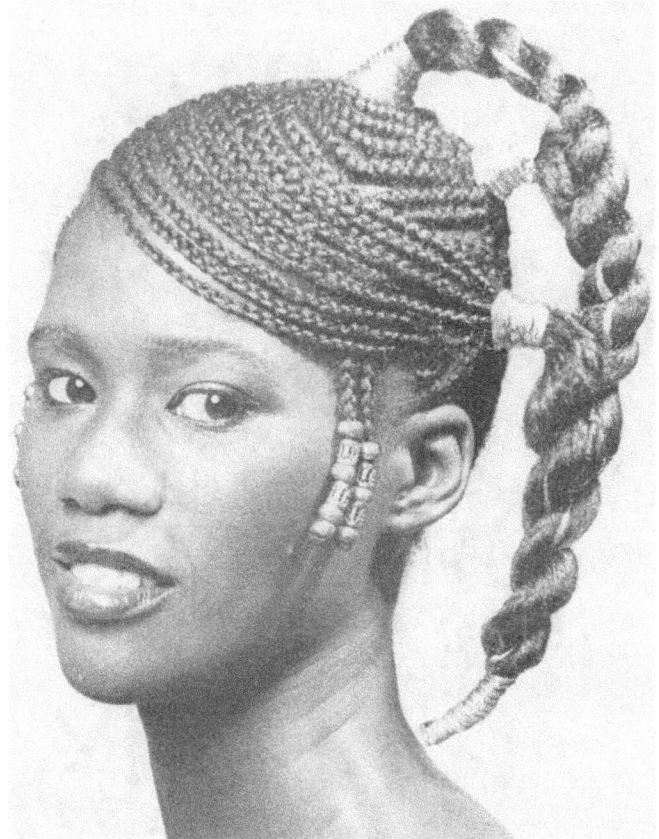

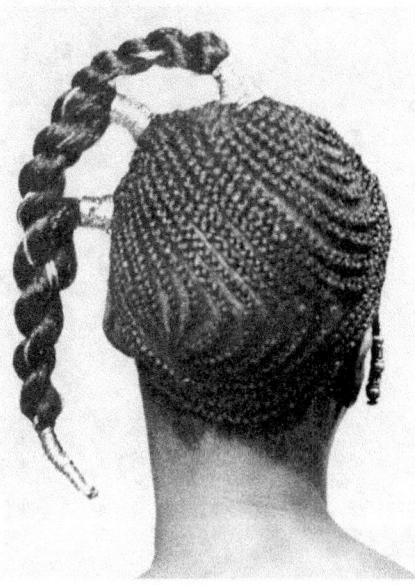

And who can object to this lovely hairdo when you are ready to take care of business? The side-swept bangs and the crown-spanning braid create a classic look. When it's time to play and let down your hair, this triple-banded twist will let everyone know you're ready to "disco"!

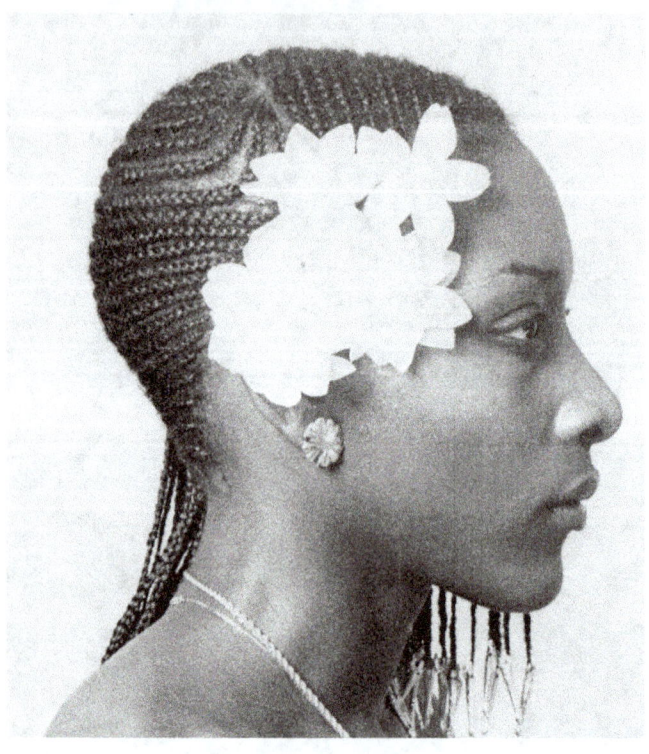

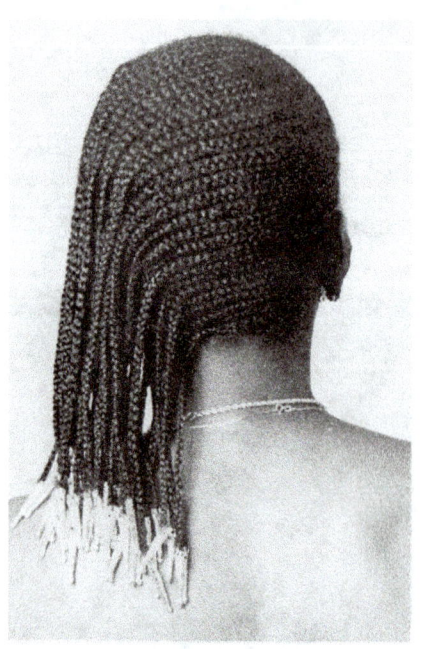

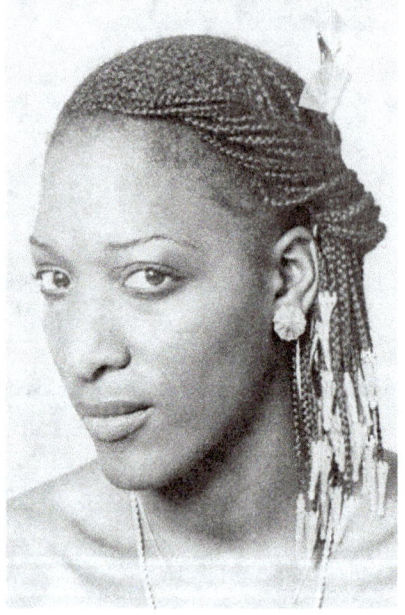

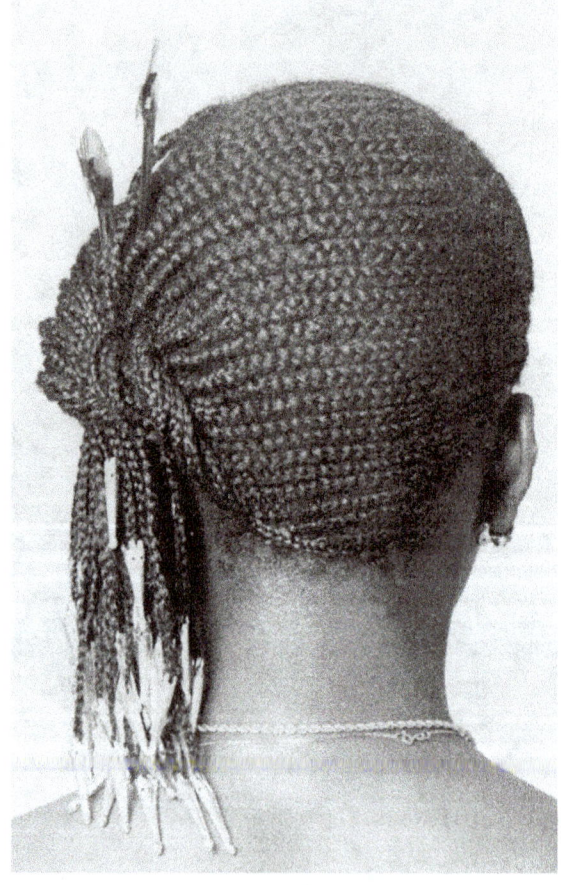

Wear flowers in your hair! This simple side-swept style will make you the center of attention. for a more sophisticated look, both front and back are rolled to meet each other. An unexpected bonus for a soft crimped effect, unbead and unbraid the hair about four inches.

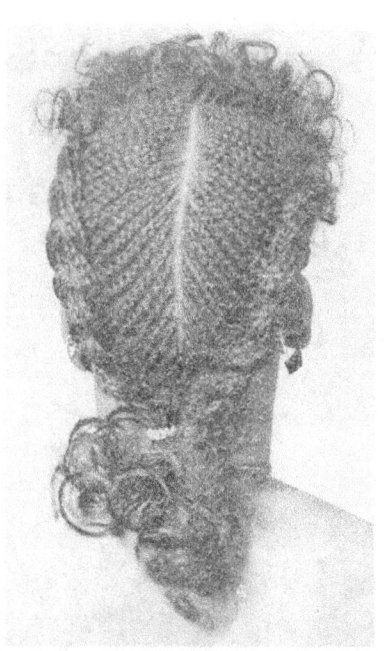

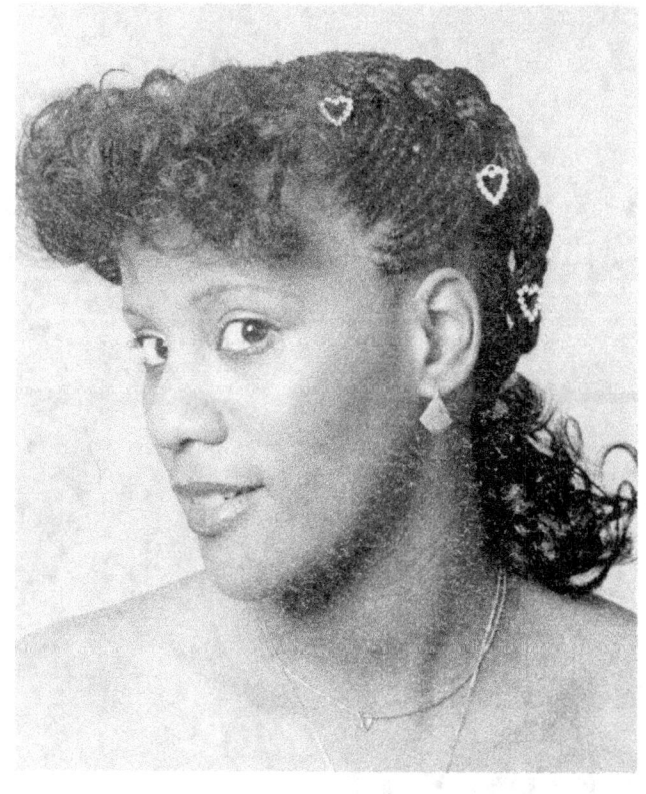

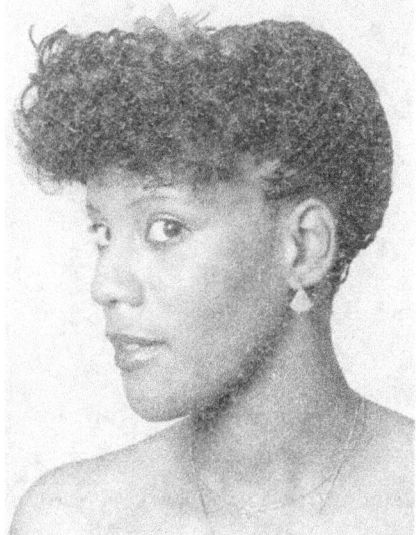

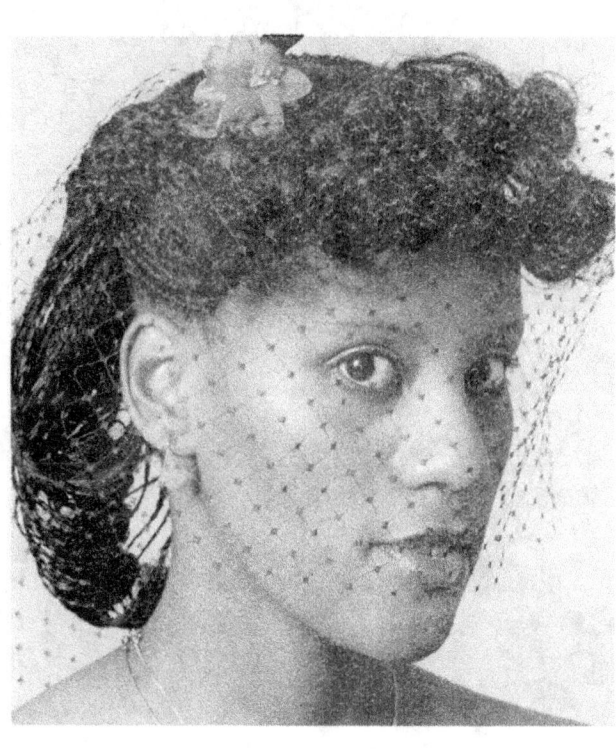

Wanda wears it whatever way she wants. This style's versatility is dependent upon the use of human hair extensions. Whether one is going to the office, shopping, school, or a formal occasion, this style works for you.

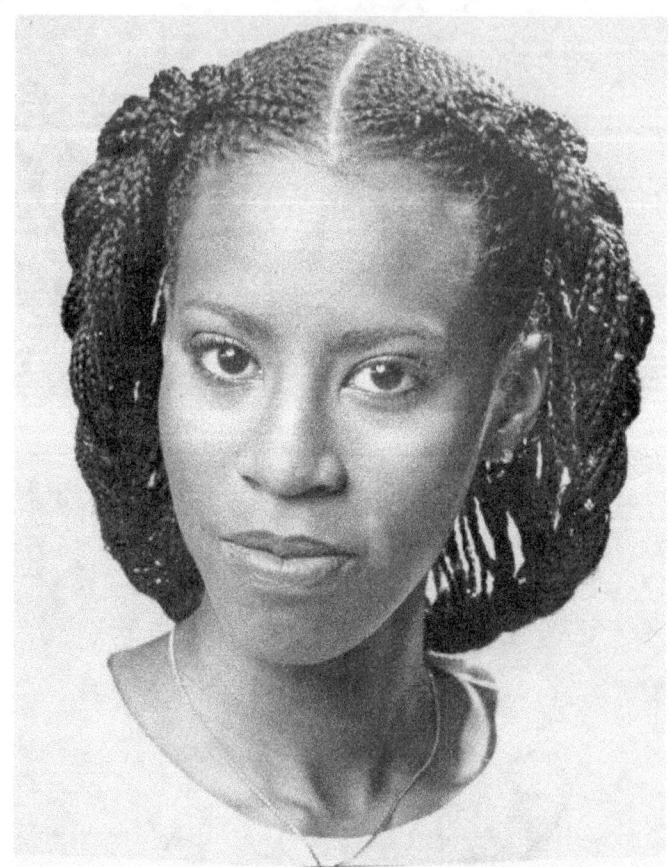

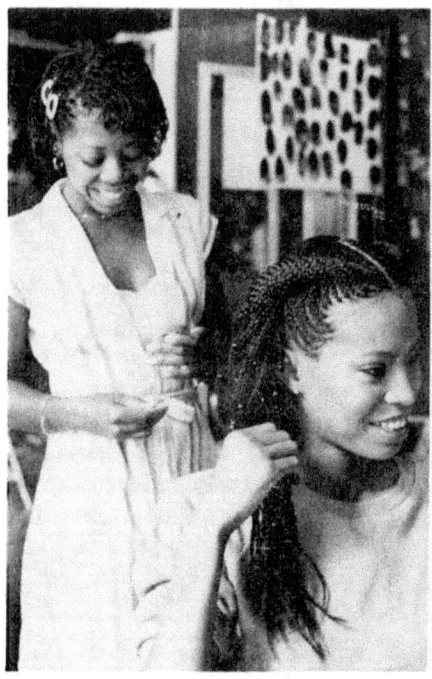

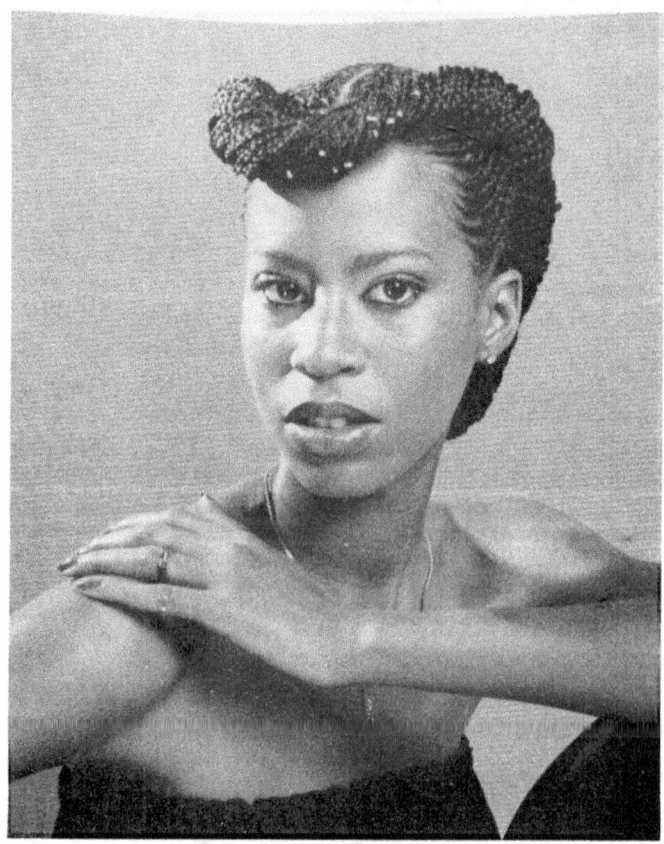

Here we are getting ready for the photo session. Kaleda's hair is being beaded. The final result is a shoulder length snood. Next, a classic by any other name . . . this head-hugging roll is a knockout! To alternate this style, roll the front back and leave the back hanging.

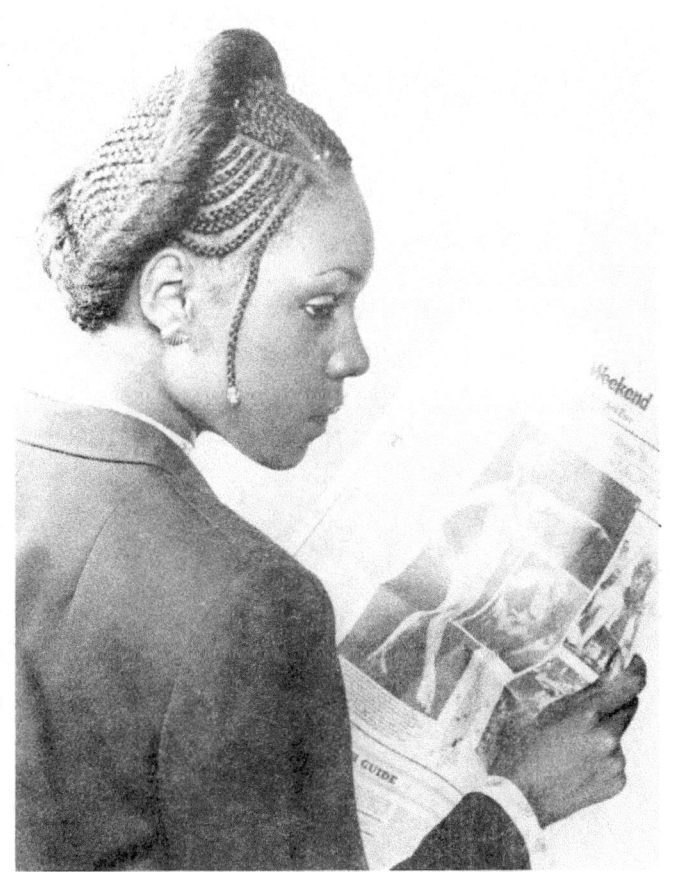

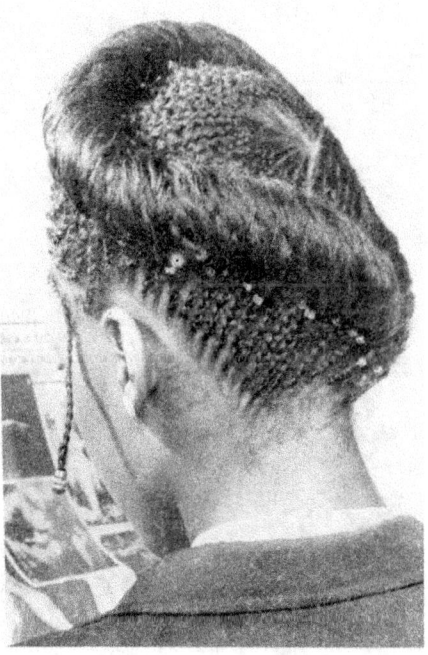

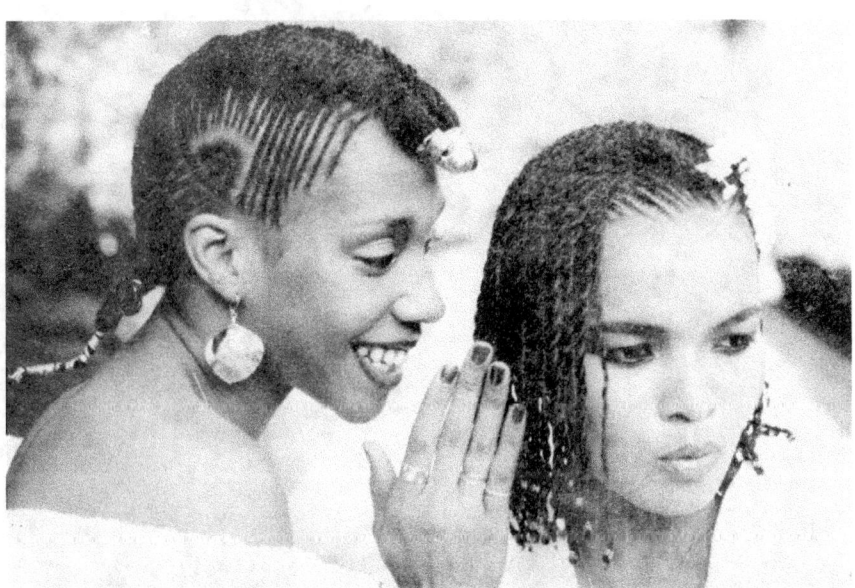

Vonnie's Style
Courtesy of Ms. Pat Wilson

Kelly and Vonnie have both got the scoop, and wouldn't you like to hear it? Vonnie's four-layered upswept style is a variation on Kaleda's style. Kelly's own hair is layered in cornrows and ends in twists. For a more contained look, both sides can be rolled back.

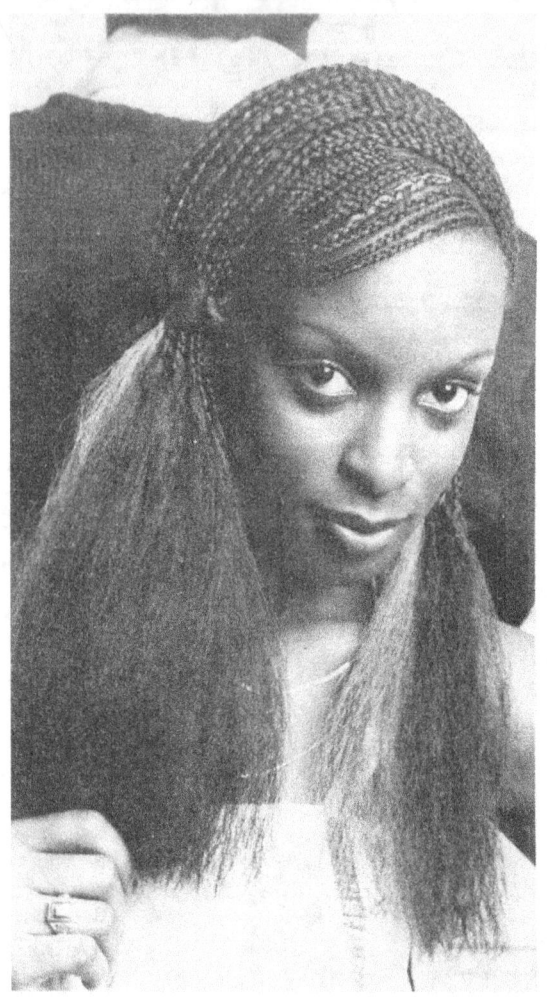

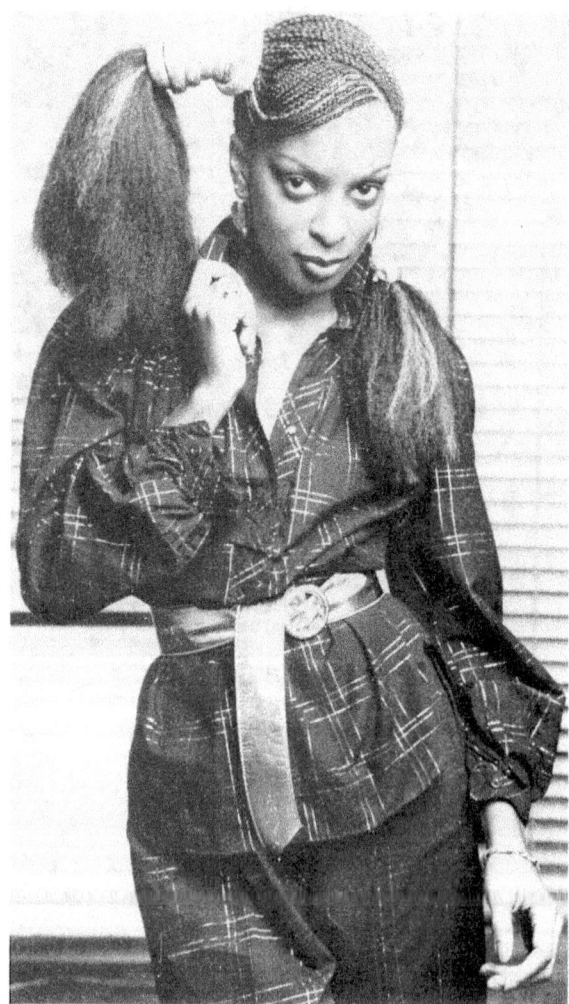

This is one fashion statement that is not likely to be overlooked. Charlotte wears a multi-layered extension style of mixed colors. The loose hair can be fashioned into rolls, twists, chignons, or whatever you can imagine.

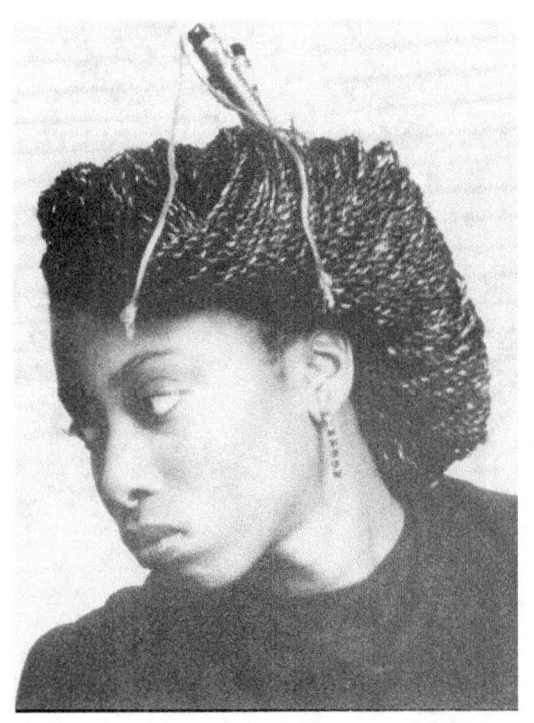

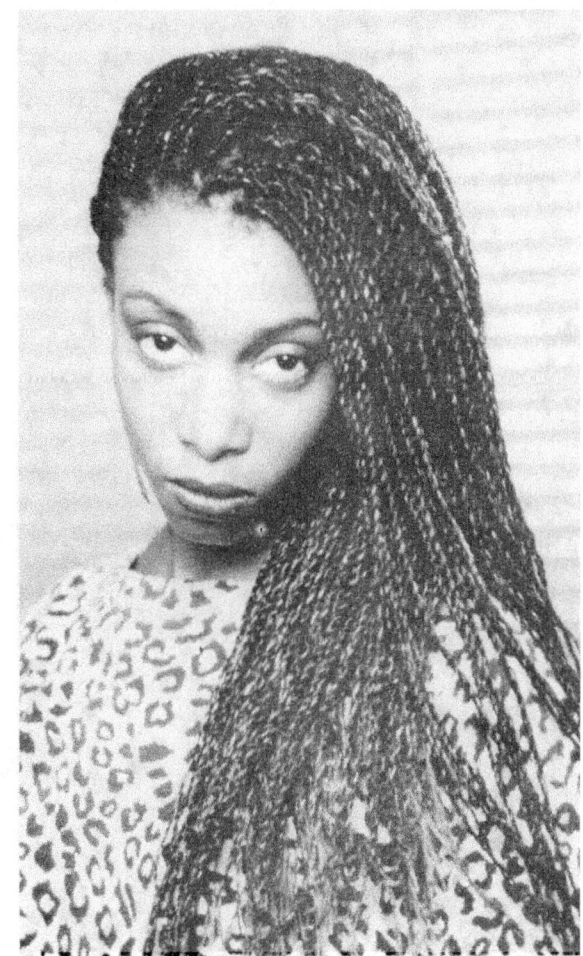

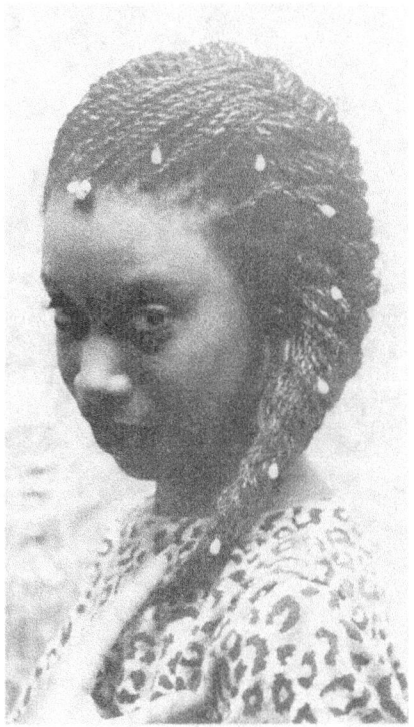

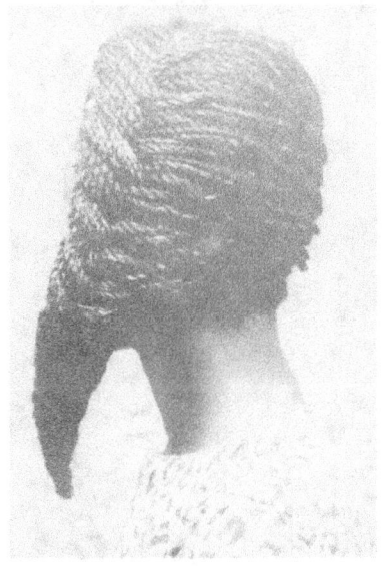

Streaks, anyone? What easier way to attain streaks than to mix black and blonde synthetic hair? Carla's twisted individual extensions adapt nicely to a variety of styles.

Style
Courtesy of Ms. Carla Brown

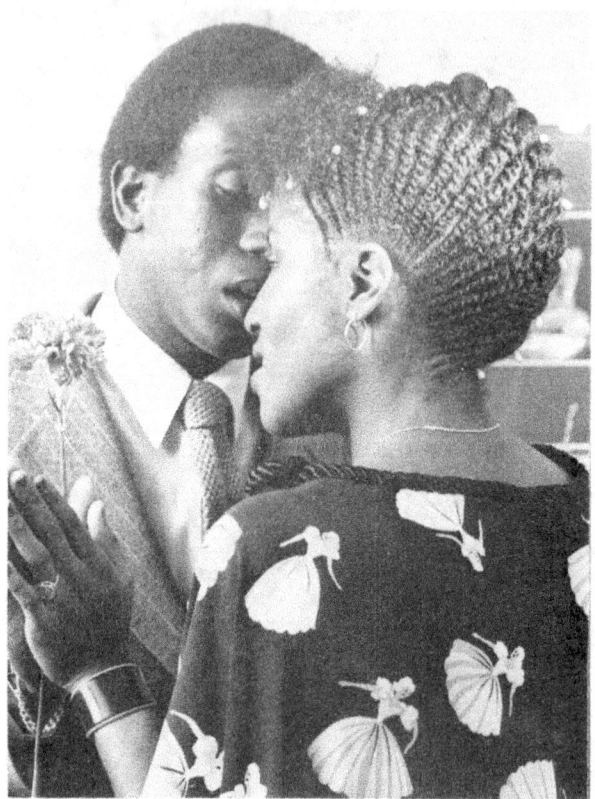

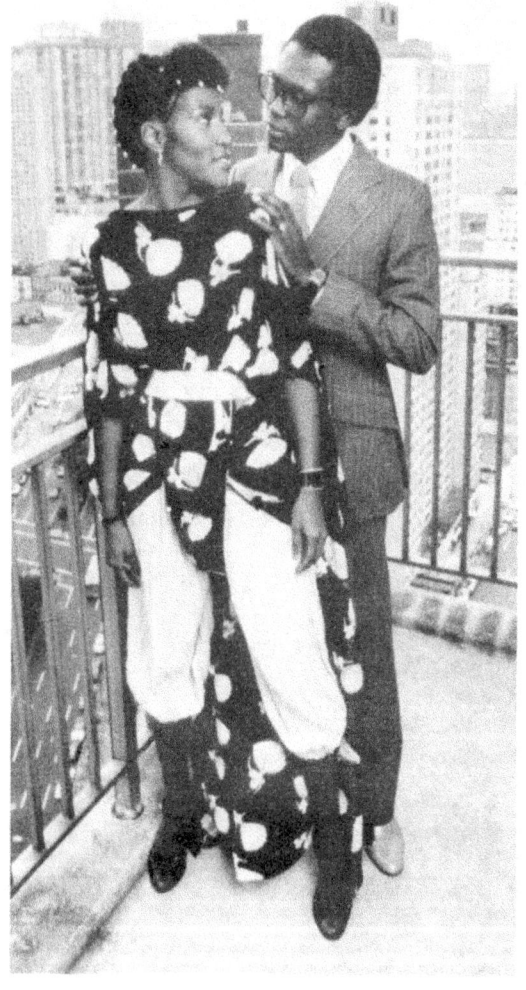

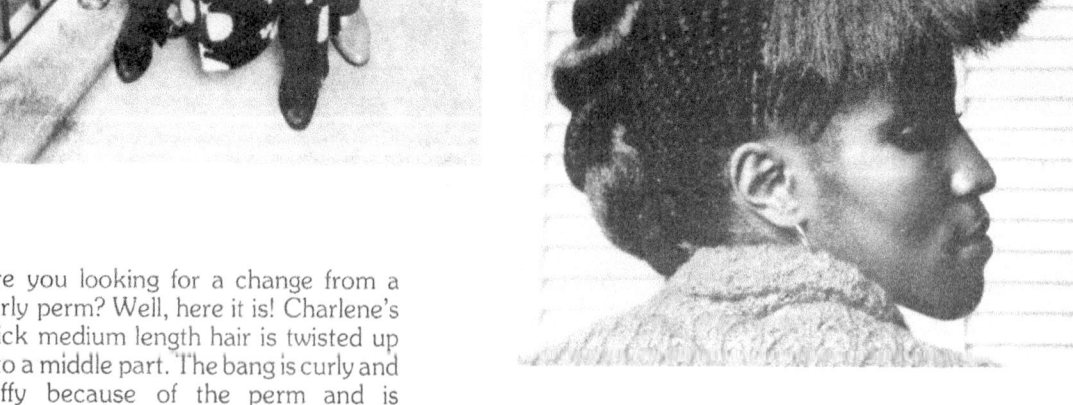

Are you looking for a change from a curly perm? Well, here it is! Charlene's thick medium length hair is twisted up into a middle part. The bang is curly and fluffy because of the perm and is encircled with pearls which proceed down the back of the head.

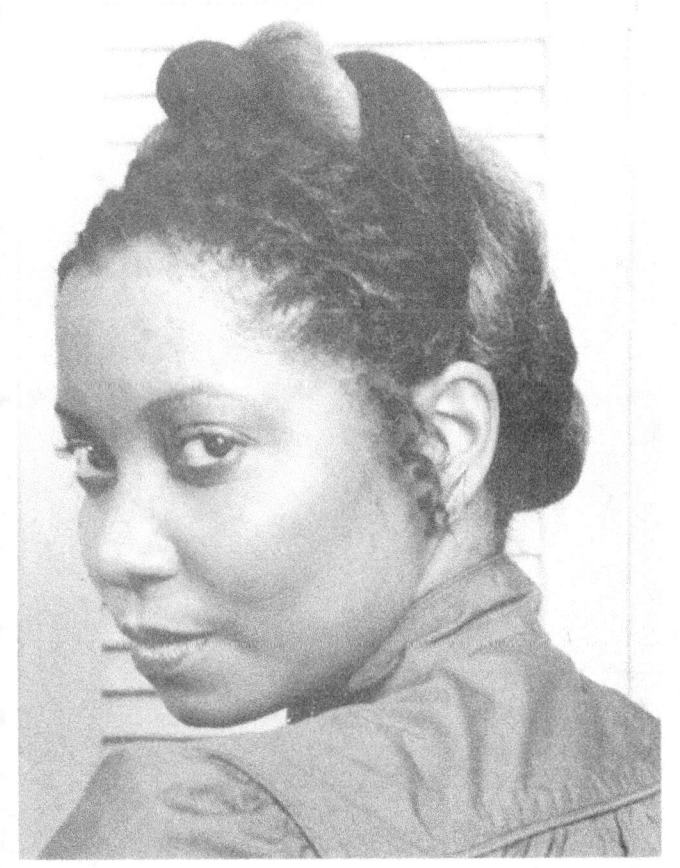

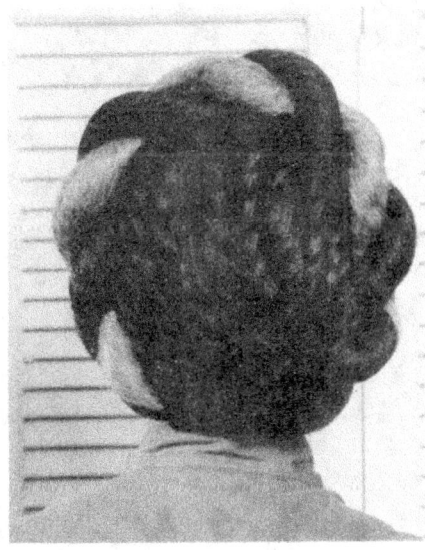

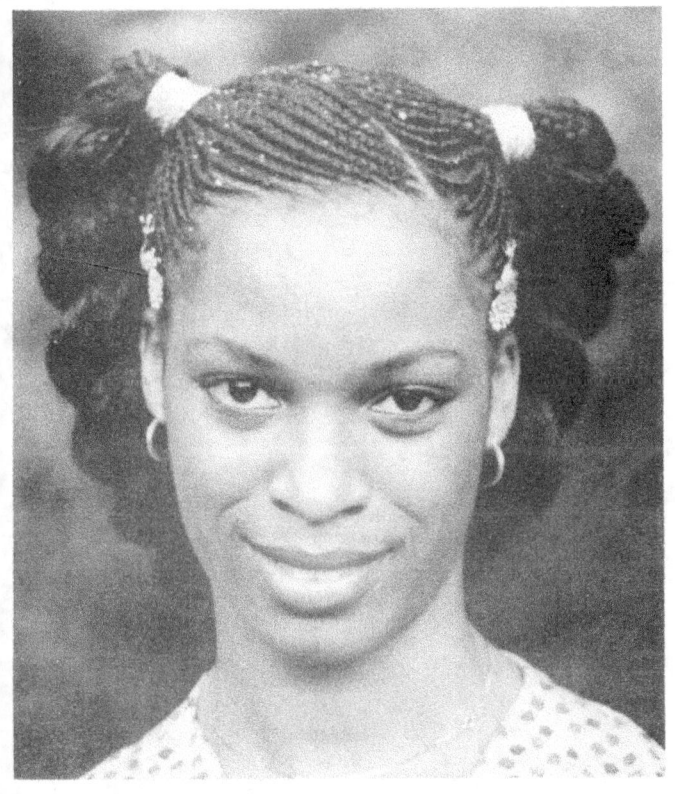

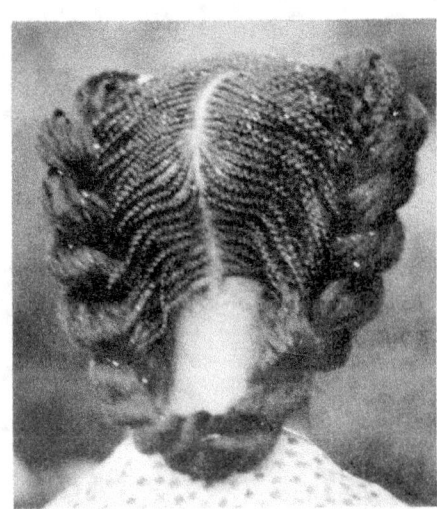

Yvonne's four-layered extension style is topped off by these face framing twists. She can also fashion two large braids in Indian style, roll or twist the hair across the crown, or wear it loose. Now, it's your turn.

23

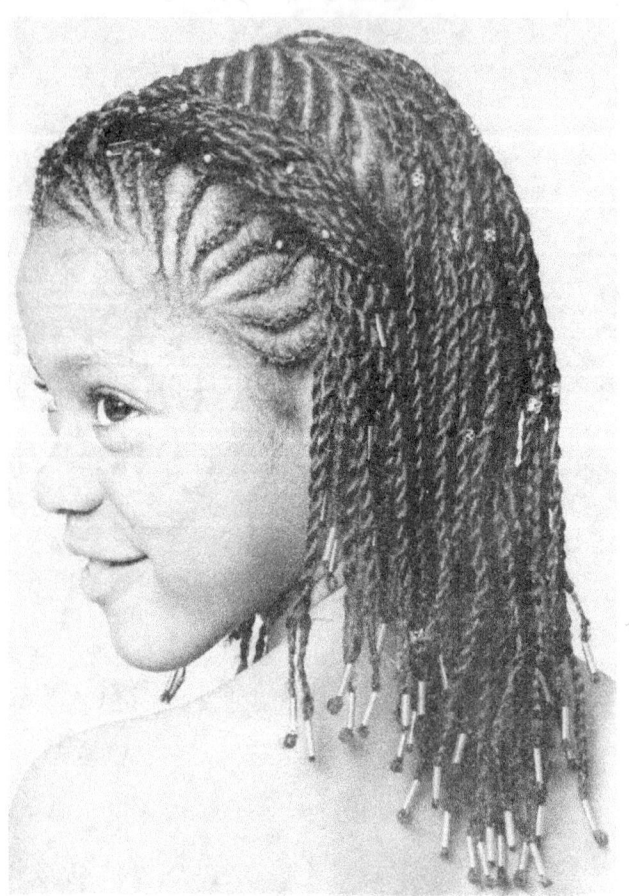

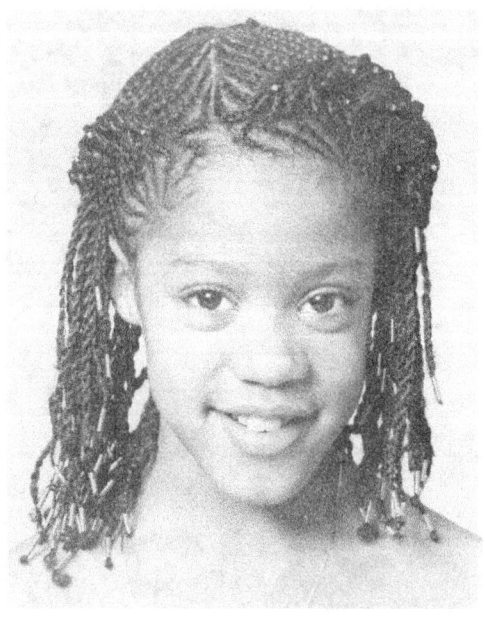

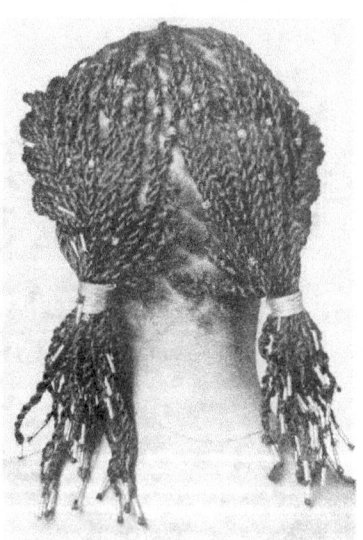

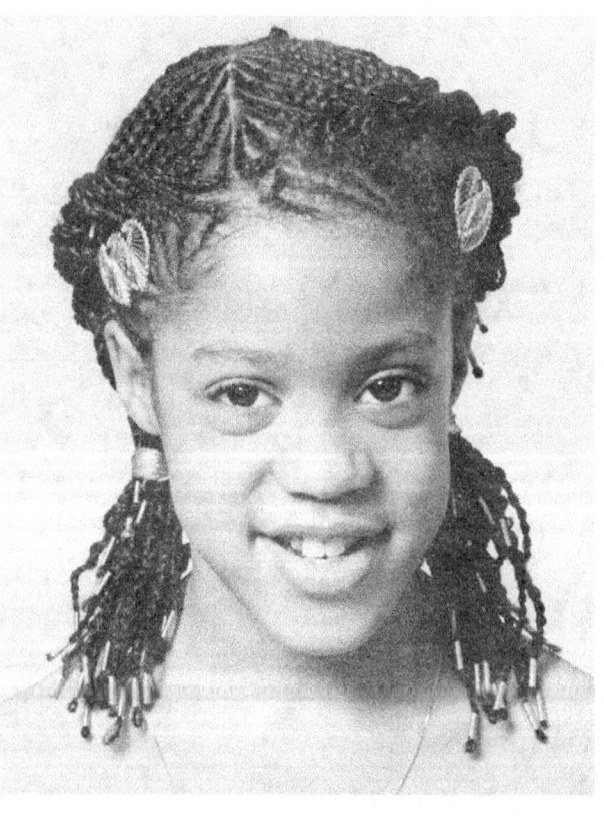

Our little star sports a style studded with beads. The front of her own hair is cornrowed in layers that end in twists. the back of her hair is done in individual twists. she can wear it in two ponytails, two rolls, two big braids, or one ponytail. This is an ideal style for the young lady with long thick hair.

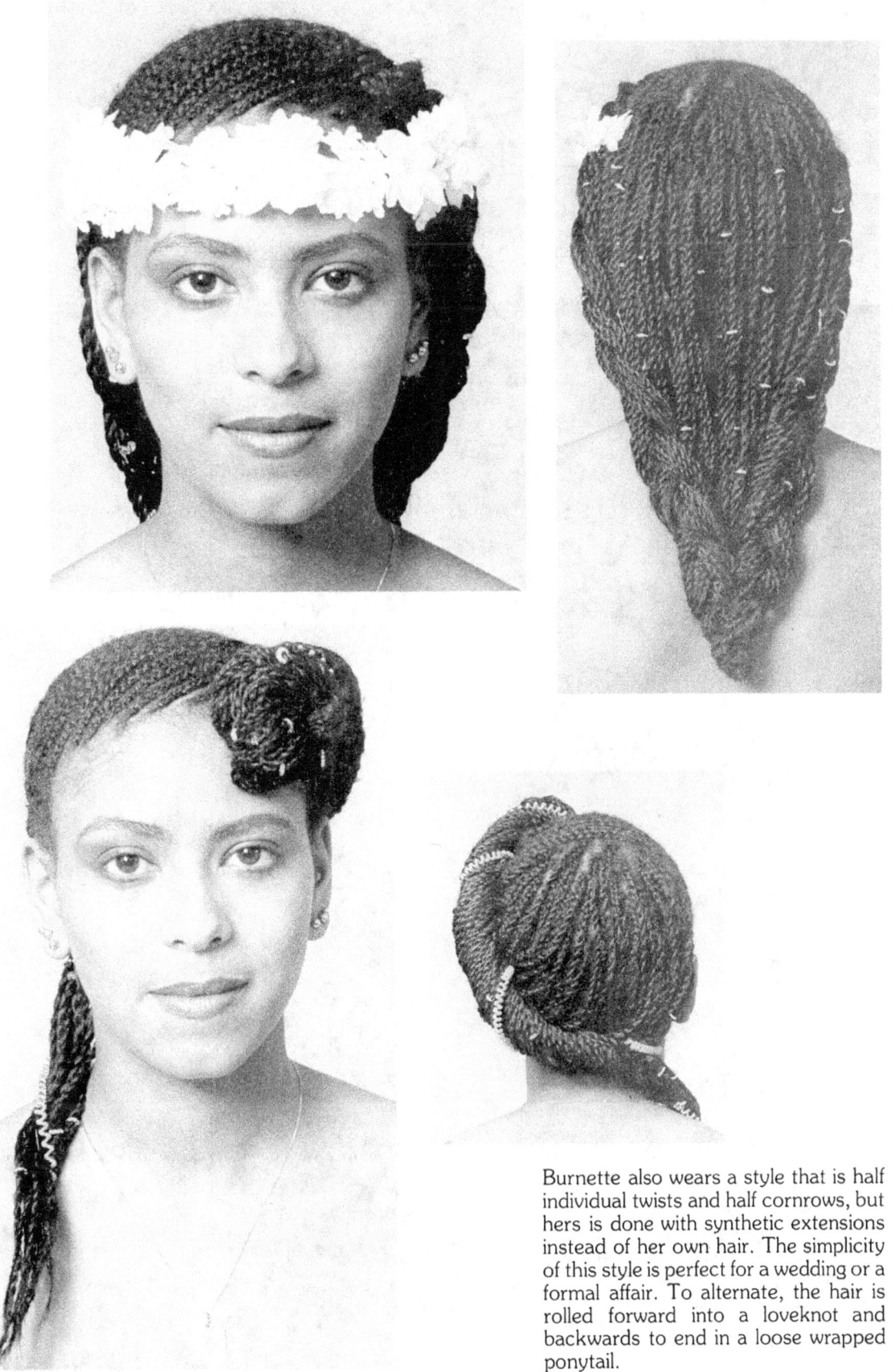

Burnette also wears a style that is half individual twists and half cornrows, but hers is done with synthetic extensions instead of her own hair. The simplicity of this style is perfect for a wedding or a formal affair. To alternate, the hair is rolled forward into a loveknot and backwards to end in a loose wrapped ponytail.

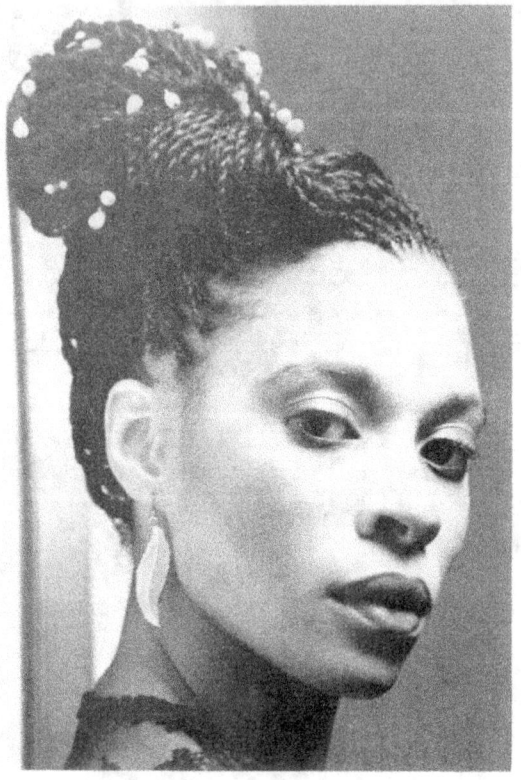

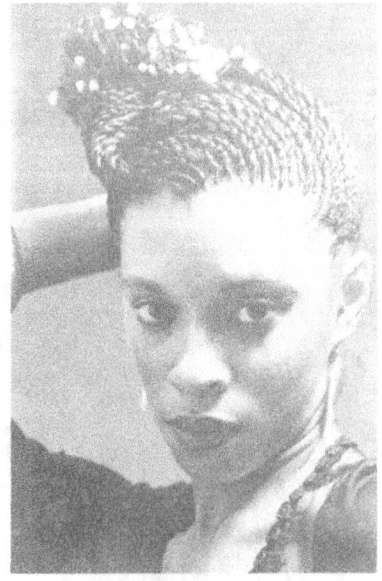

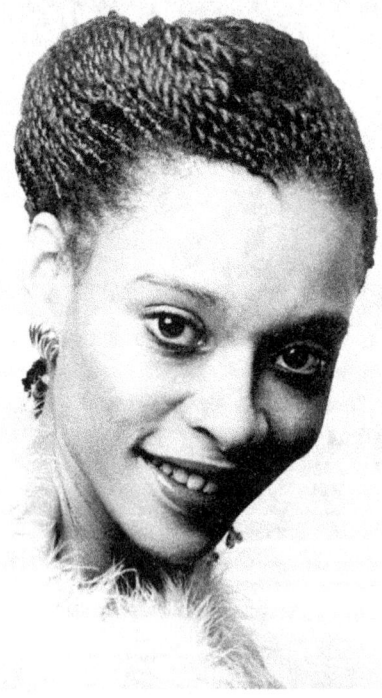

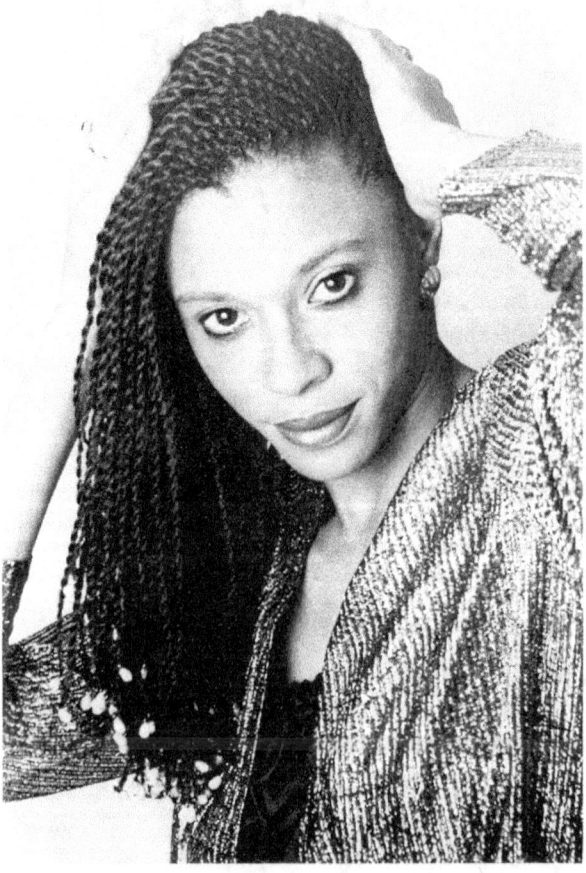

Darnella's style consists of cornrowed and individual twists. For a formal look, the hair is piled on the side of the head. The second style is softly rolled to the back of the head, and the third hangs freely. A ponytail or a large braid can also alter this style's appearance.

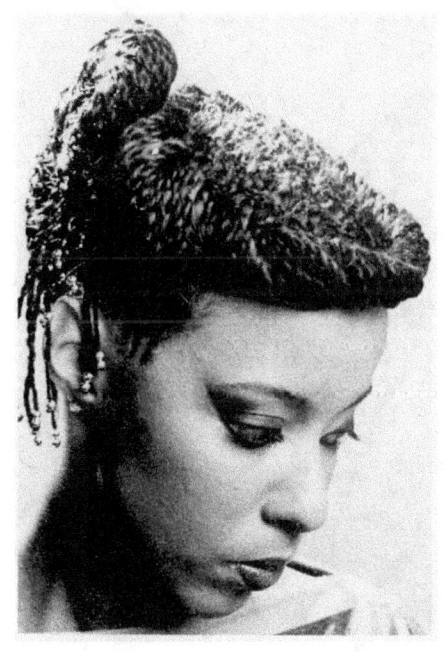

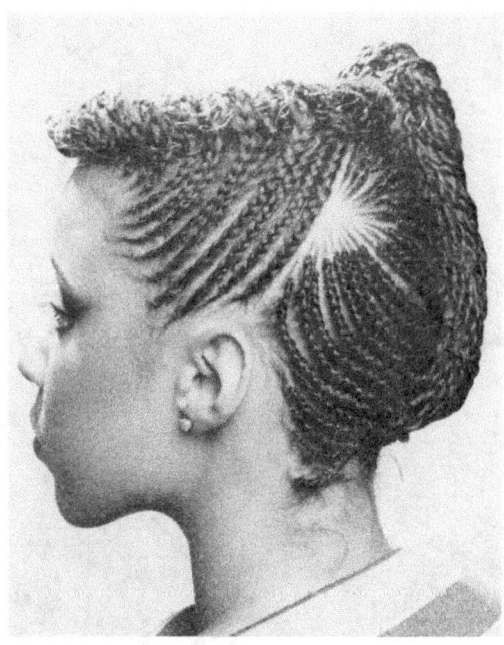

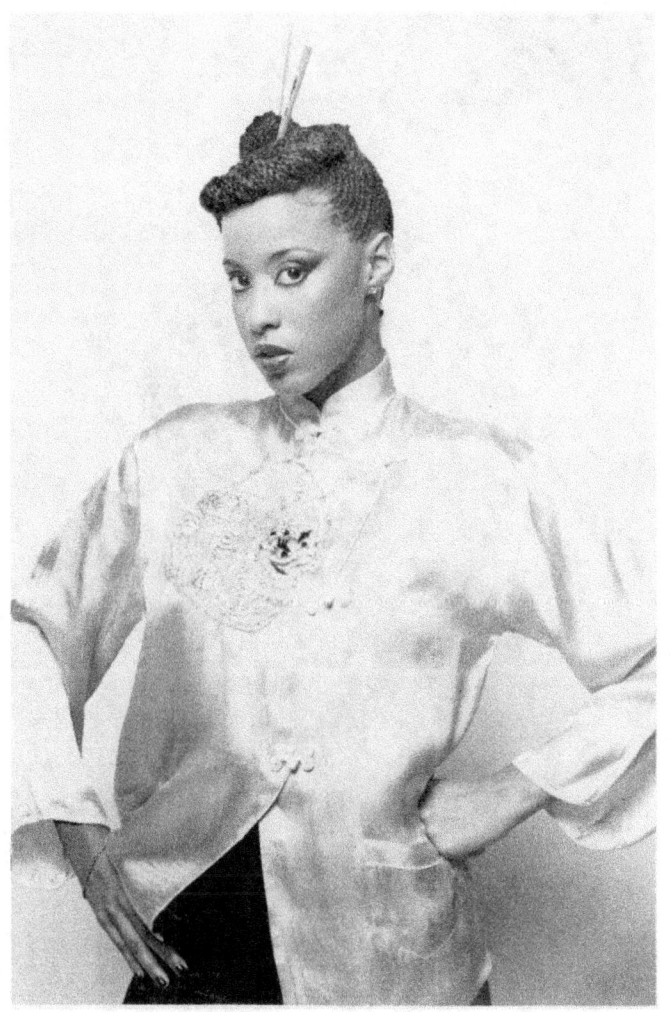

Ah, the inscrutable one is here! Zaida wears a double-rolled style that is topped in a basket weave. The back is twisted at the ends and meets the top roll which also ends in twists before being rolled. A sunburst pattern draws the eye to the side back. The back roll can also be let down.

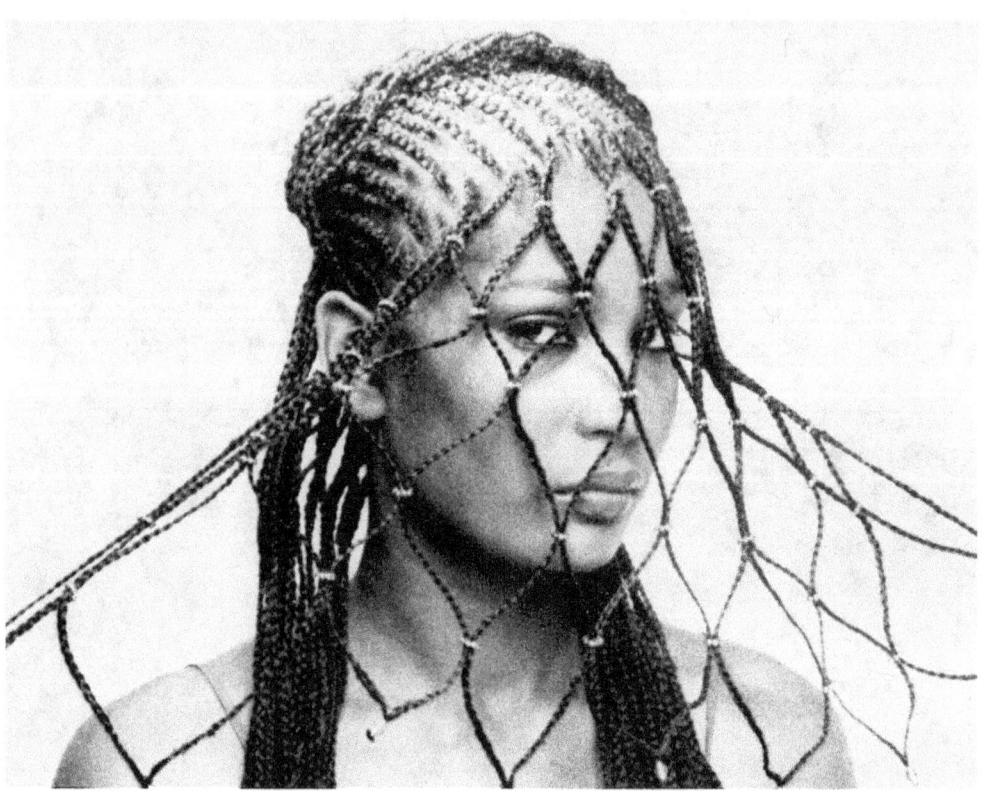

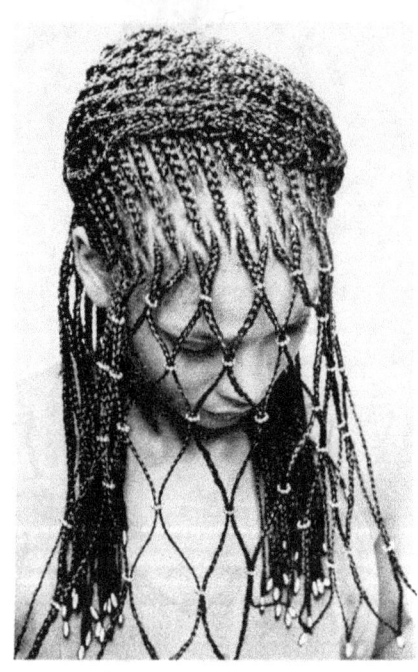

Ooh, la la! You'll be the talk of the town in this one! Glenda wears a braided beaded veil, topped by a basket weave beret. All the hanging braids were beaded. And no, she doesn't wear it like that all of the time. The veil can be pulled back and secured to elicit a halo effect. The crimped look also adds variety.

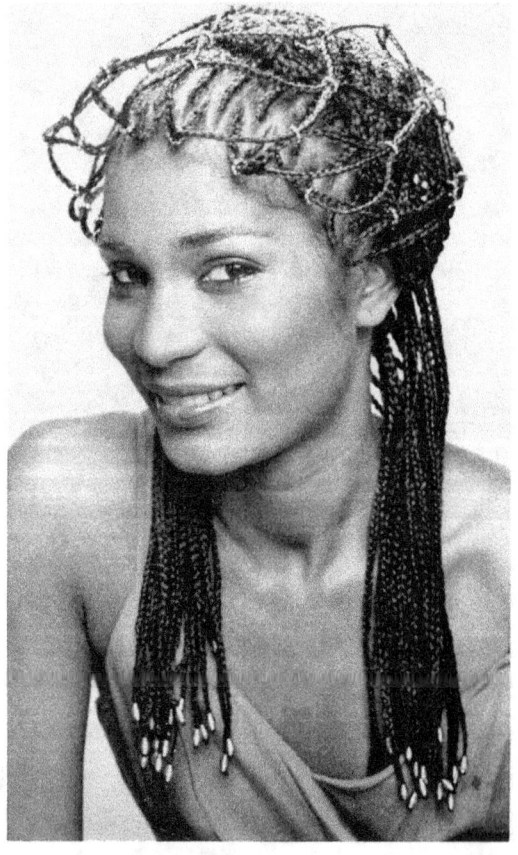

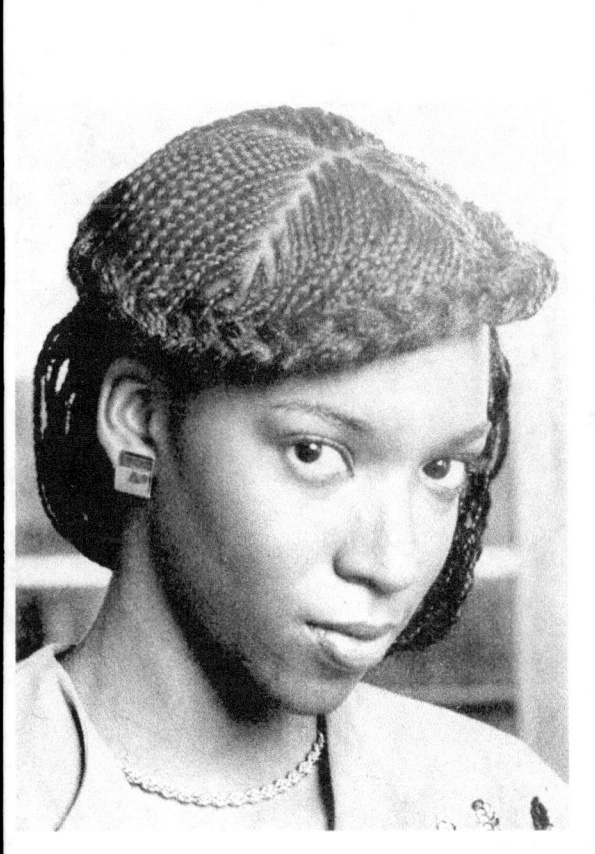

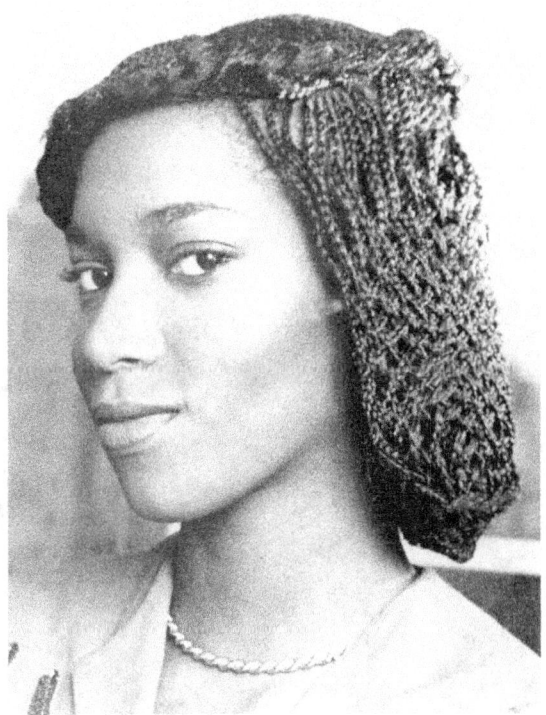

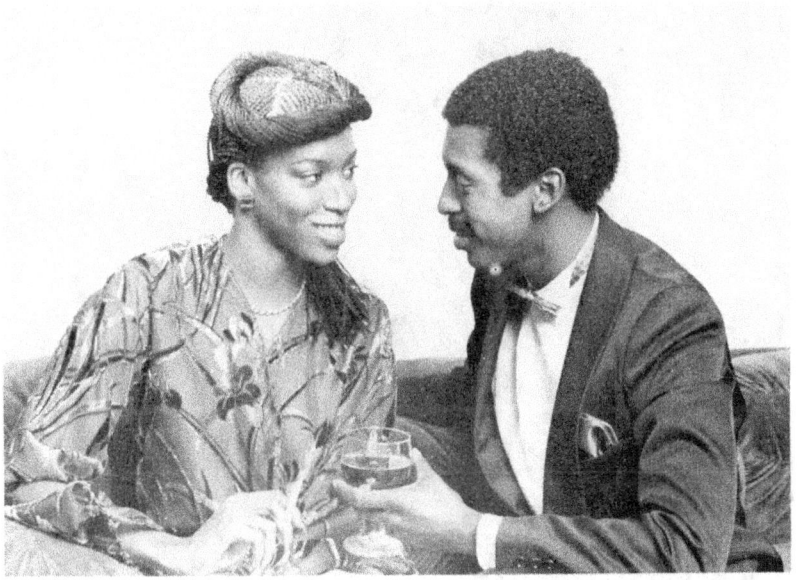

For those of us who love hats . . . here's to you! Jeri wears her "designer" hat on top of a woven braided net. For the admiring eyes of the man in her life, the crown is rolled and ends are twisted.

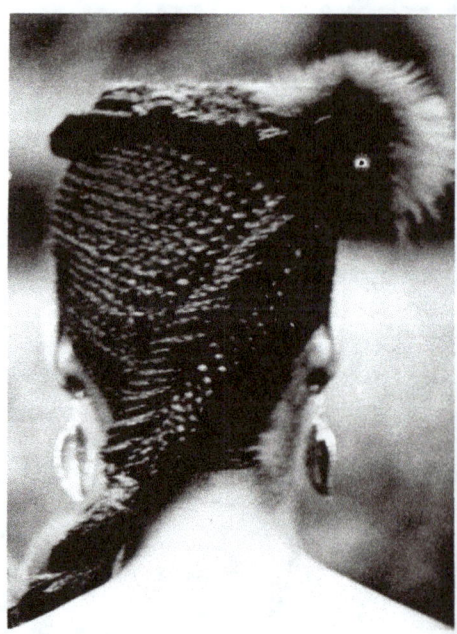

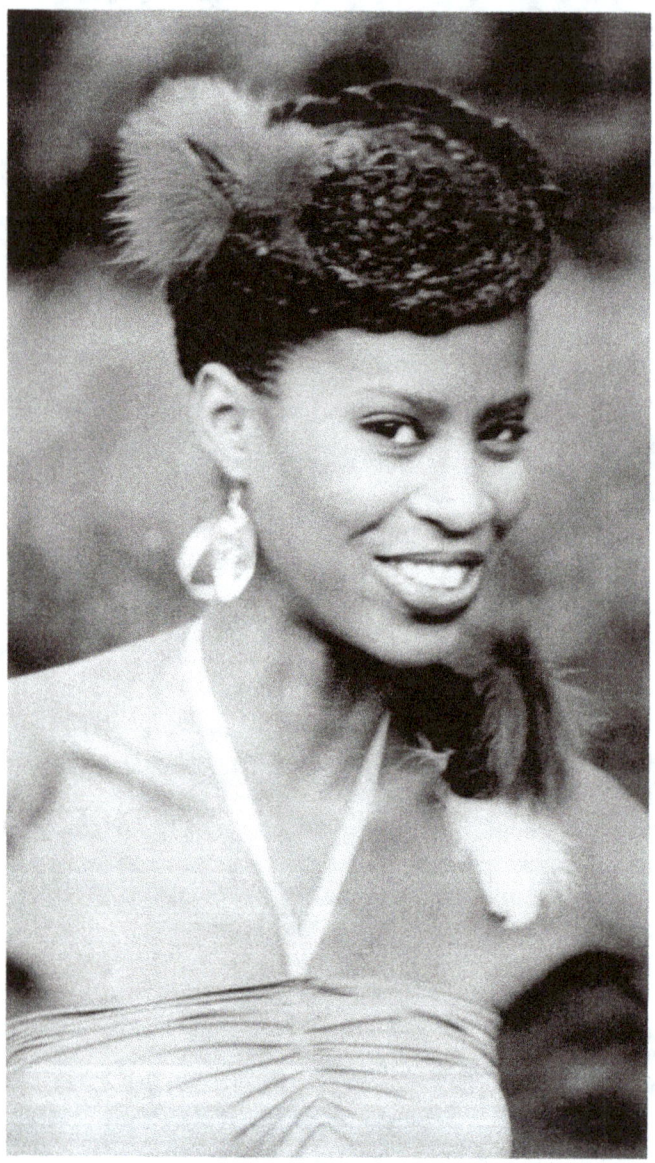

Hats off to . . . well, this hat isn't really removable. It's a basket weave and is the crowning glory to a closely braided extension cornrow style. The back is set off by a double-rolled braid. There's nothing like a feather in your cap, so why not three?

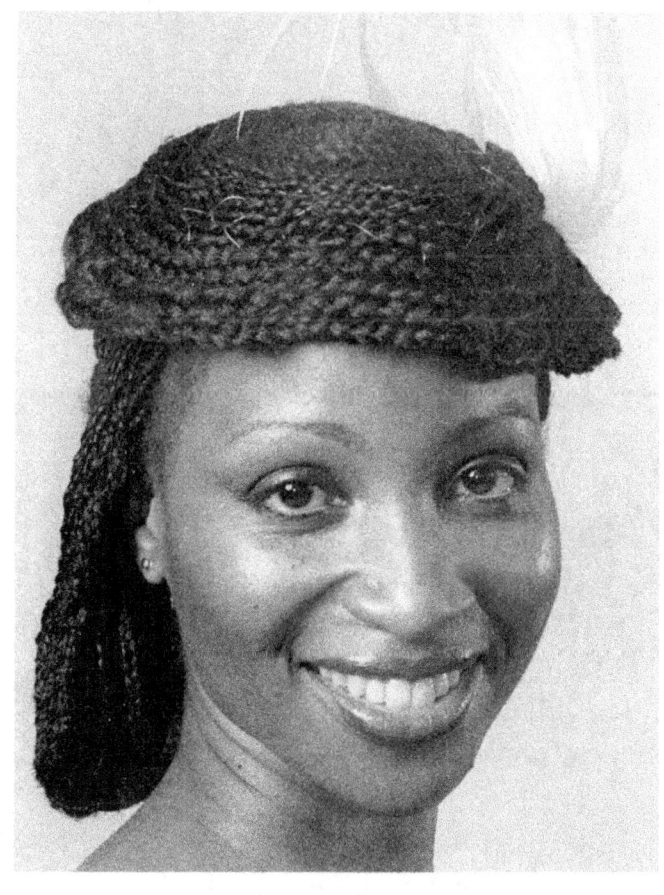

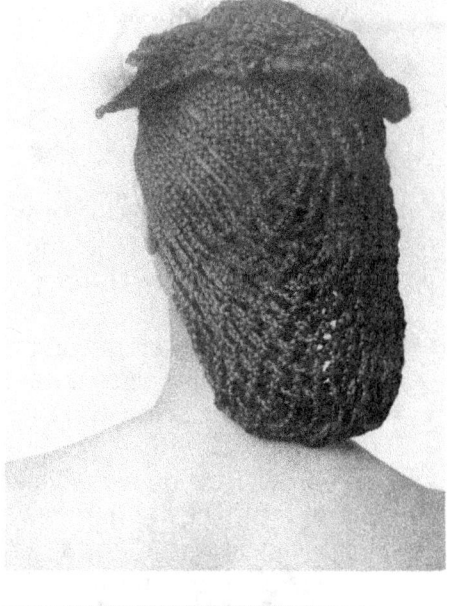

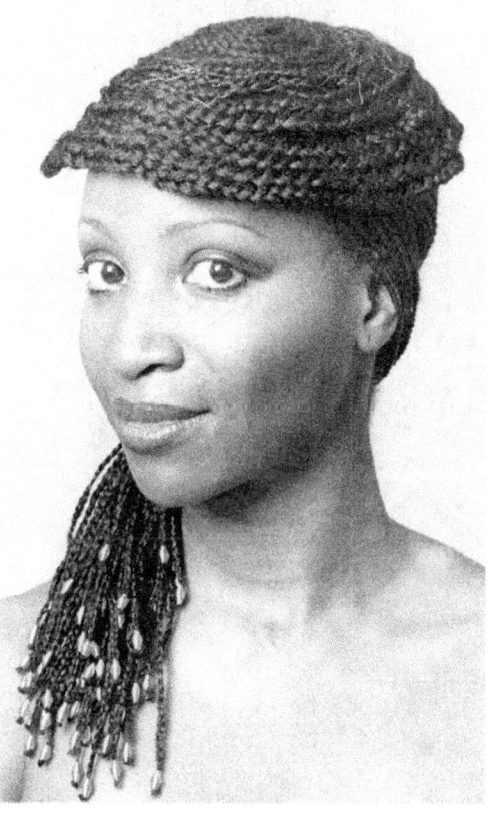

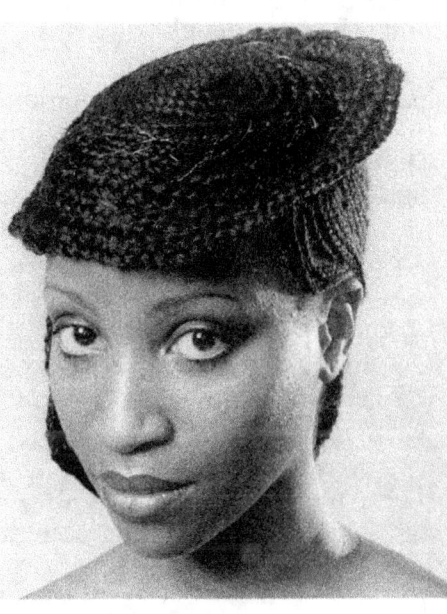

Once again, we have a variation on a theme. Phyllis' hat is a circular with an upturned brim. When not wearing the "net", she sports a beaded ponytail or lets the hair hang free.

BRAID CARE

- Get off to a good start by first washing the hair and then deep conditioning it.

- Oil your scalp before braiding your hair. The oil will be distributed along the hair shaft during brushing, and oil need not be put on the hair.

- If you have a hard time managing your hair, you may want to use a blow out comb before braiding.

- Be sure that your hair is not braided too tightly because headaches and/or scalp bumps could result. The time that you save by wearing braids should be pain-free.

- In order to keep your braids neat as long as possible, tie the head up in a scarf or stocking cap (remember them?) every night. A hairpin or two at the nape of the neck will keep it in place.

- When braids start getting fuzzy, dip a cloth into hot water, wring it out gently, and place it over your head until it cools. The steam will draw up the stray ends.

- The hair can be washed while it is in braids. Wearing a stocking cap, first wet the hair, spread shampoo on the hands, and gently massage it into the scalp. Rinse the hair thoroughly, at least three times. A hot oil treatment will reduce dandruff and dryness of the scalp. Finish up with a no-rinse conditioner.

- Hair breakage is held to a minimum while the hair is in braids, but the normal shedding and regrowth cycle of the hair is not. Therefore, do not be alarmed at the amount of hair that is shed when you take out the braids.

  WARNING: If braids are left in too long, the hair will lock at the roots and the detangling process may cause excessive damage.

- Upon taking braids out, always comb out each section as you undo it. Using plastic bristles, brush the whole head thoroughly before washing.

- If you are using extensions, upon removal you must unbraid them all the way to the starting point in order to avoid pulling out your own hair.

- All textures of hair (whether permed, pressed, or natural) can benefit from being braided. The hair gets a much needed rest, and the hair shaft is protected against constant picking and combing.

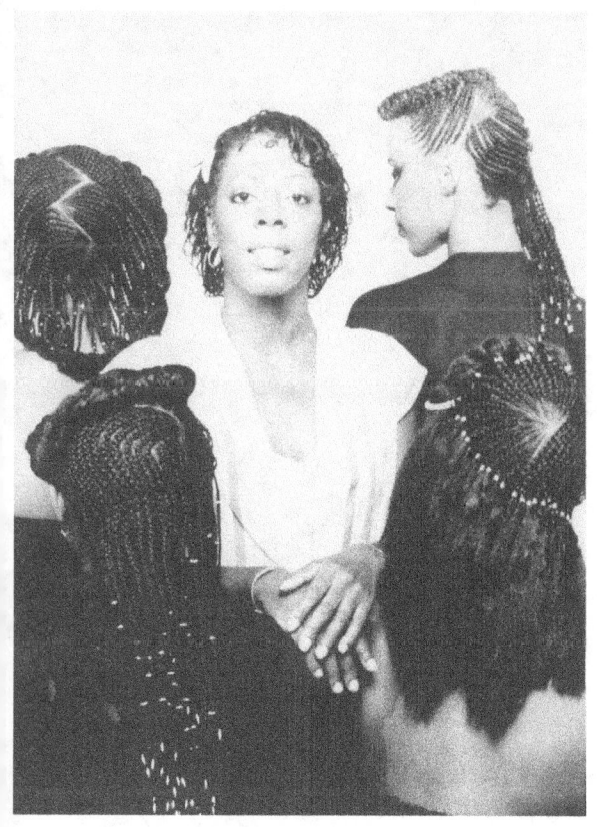

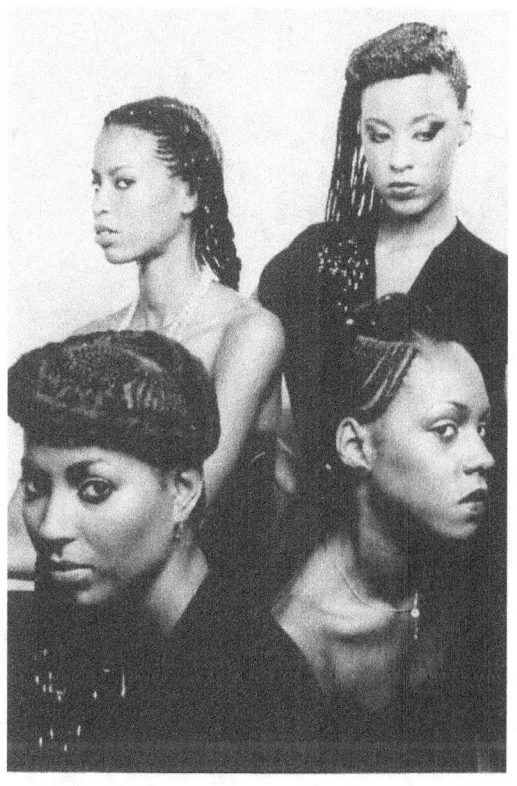

CREDITS

Many thanks to all the models who sat so still for so long.

Special acknowledgment to Drs. Shirley and Karl Leone. Thank you for caring.

Photographers
Kwame Brathwaite
Gene Ward

Book Design
Richard Waller